Natural Killer Cells - Lessons and Challenges

Edited by Leisheng Zhang

Published in London, United Kingdom

Natural Killer Cells - Lessons and Challenges
http://dx.doi.org/10.5772/intechopen.105658
Edited by Leisheng Zhang

Contributors
Leisheng Zhang, Zhihai Han, Zhongchao Han, Xiaoming Feng, Vida Homayouni, Fariba Dehghan, Roya Sherkat, Li Zhang, Chang Liu, Chang-Sheng Shao, Xin Yu, Ya-Hui Wu, Qing Huang, Shixun Ma, Li Li, Hui Cai, Tiankang Guo, Jintang Yin, Xiaohu Wang, Chongya Yang

First published in London, United Kingdom, 2023 by IntechOpen
IntechOpen is the global imprint of INTECHOPEN LIMITED, registered in England and Wales, registration number: 11086078, 5 Princes Gate Court, London, SW7 2QJ, United Kingdom

British Library Cataloguing-in-Publication Data
A catalogue record for this book is available from the British Library

Additional hard and PDF copies can be obtained from orders@intechopen.com

Natural Killer Cells - Lessons and Challenges
Edited by Leisheng Zhang
p. cm.
Print ISBN 978-1-83768-480-9
Online ISBN 978-1-83768-481-6
eBook (PDF) ISBN 978-1-83768-482-3

Meet the editor

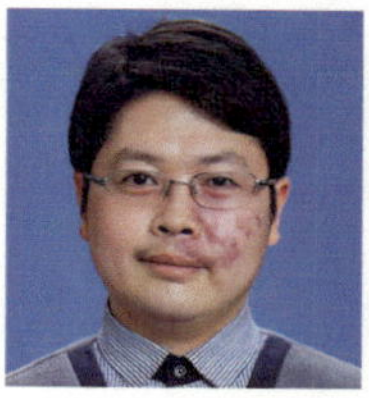

Professor Leisheng Zhang is a cell biologist and the leader of a research team devoted to tissue engineering and regenerative medicine. In 2012, he obtained a BVetMed from Jilin University, China. In 2018, he obtained a Ph.D. in Cellular Biology from the Chinese Academy of Medical Sciences & Peking Union Medical College (CAMS & PUMC) and Tsinghua University, China. In 2019 and 2022, Dr. Zhang conducted post-doctoral research at the Nankai University School of Medicine and the Chinese Academy of Sciences (CAS). He has worked on projects for the National Natural Science Foundation of China and has published more than sixty articles, thirteen books, and more than thirty patents.

Contents

Preface

Natural killer (NK) cells, also known as innate lymphoid cells (ILCs), belong to ILCs with broad distributions in the body. NK cells encompass distinct populations based on CD56 intensity in humans and CD11b and CD27 expression in mice. NK cells are unique immune cells that are capable of efficient killing of transformed and infected cells as well as pathogenic microorganisms and tumor cells. As such, autologous and allogeneic NK cells have advantages in cancer immunotherapy, delaying aging, and eradicating pathogenic infections.

For decades, investigators in the field have identified NK cells from a variety of sources, such as peripheral blood, umbilical cord blood, placental blood, NK cell lines, and even stem cells. Of these, perinatal blood-derived NK cells have proven to exhibit robust ex vivo expansion activity and thus have greater potential for use in cancer immunosurveillance and immunotherapy compared to their counterparts. Currently, NK cell-based immunotherapy has been demonstrated to be safe and effective for treating cancers including hematologic malignancies and metastatic solid tumors via antibody-dependent cell-mediated cytotoxicity (ADCC), granule enzymes, and perforin dispenses with pre-sensitization and antigen presentation. The effectiveness of NK cells in the elimination and surveillance of cancers has fascinated immunologists for decades.

This book discusses NK cell-based cytotherapy and highlights NK cells as essential components of the innate immune system and tumor immune surveillance. Distinct from chimeric antigen receptor-transduced T (CAR-T) cells, NK cells or CAR-transduced NK (CAR-NK) cells are exempt from untoward effects such as neurotoxicity, cytokine storm syndrome (CSS), and graft-versus-host disease (GvHD). As a pivotal part of the innate immune system, NK cells have been recognized as an attractive option for cancer immunotherapy due to their ability to kill cancer cells or infected cells without prior sensitization. Collectively, NK cells are unique cell sources with anti-neoplastic, anti-infectious, and immunomodulatory effects based on both direct cellular cytotoxicity and cytokine production that is not major histocompatibility complex (MHC) restricted. It is noteworthy that NK cells have been reported with the capability of killing tumor cells autonomously in the tumor microenvironment, which thus represents the unique effect against immune escape, tumor progression, and metastasis. Overall, this book highlights the feasibility of NK cell-based cytotherapy for cancer immunotherapy and the promising prospects of NK cells or CAR-NK cells in regenerative medicine in the future, which will benefit the development of cancer immunosurveillance and cancer immunotherapy.

Leisheng Zhang
Chinese Academy of Medical Sciences & Peking Union Medical Colleage
(CAMS & PUMC),
Tianjin, China

Section 1

The Landscape of Natural Killer Cells

Chapter 1

Natural Killer Cells for Cancer Immunotherapy: Opportunities and Challenges

Leisheng Zhang, Xiaoming Feng, Zhihai Han and Zhongchao Han

Abstract

Natural killer (NK) cells are advantaged immune cells and play a pivotal role in both innate and adaptive immune responses. To date, autogenous and allogenic NK cells have been generated from a variety of origins, including perinatal blood (e.g., umbilical cord blood and placental blood), peripheral blood, and even stem cells (hematopoietic stem cells and pluripotent stem cells). NK cells function mainly *via* antibody-dependent cell-mediated cytotoxicity (ADCC), direct cytolytic effect, and paracrine effects (e.g., IFN-γ, GM-CSF, granzyme, and perforin). Distinguishing from the adaptive immunizing cells (e.g., T and B lymphocytes), NK cells, and chimeric antigen receptor-transduced NK (CAR-NK), cell-based cytotherapy is adequate to fulfill the biofunction of eliminating pathogenic infection, combating hematological malignancies and metastatic solid tumors, and delaying aging. In this chapter, we mainly focus on the state-of-the-art renewal of NK cell-based cytotherapy for cancer immunosurveillance and immunotherapy from the view of high-efficient *in vitro* preparation (e.g., candidate cell sources and *ex vivo* cultivation) and preclinical and clinical investigation. Furthermore, we also figure out the promising prospects and the concomitant challenges of NK cell-based remedies for cancer management in future, which will collectively benefit the development of NK cell-based cancer immunotherapy in future.

Keywords: natural killer cells, cancer immunotherapy, CAR-NK cells, preclinical and clinical investigation

1. Introduction

Cancer, including hematological malignancies and metastatic solid tumors, is one of the leading causes of death worldwide with increasing incidence and mortality, which has thus become a major public health issue and heavy burden to patients and their families [1, 2]. For example, a total of over 4,568,000 cases were newly diagnosed cancer in China, and over 3,002,000 cancer deaths occurred in 2020 [3]. Of them, lung cancer is the most frequent type, followed by colorectal cancer and gastric cancer, whereas lung cancer, hepatocellular carcinoma, and stomach cancers are the top three most deadly subtypes of cancers in the general population.

For decades, depicting the cancer pattern has also been acknowledged to provide basic know-hows for developing novel strategies for cancer management [4, 5]. To date, a variety of modifiable risk factors for cancer have been identified to fuel the shift of cancer transition, such as oncogenes, air pollution, smoking, alcohol consumption, unhealthful dietary habits, obesity, physical inactivity, infectious agents, diabetes, improved livelihood, and even rapid economic development [6–8]. For example, cancer-related fatigue is one of the most distressing and prevalent symptoms among patients, which usually results in great research challenges [9].

For decades, effective implementation strategies have been developed to optimize the advancements in the fields of tumor survivorship, diagnosis, treatment, and end-of-life care [10]. For instance, a series of treatments have been developed to conquer cancers with high uncontrolled cell division and heterogeneity, including surgery (e.g., laparoscopic rectal surgery and robotic surgery) [11, 12], photothermal therapy (PTT) [13–15], radiotherapy [16], chemotherapy [17], oncolytic virotherapy [18], RNA vaccine [19, 20], hormone therapy [21], peptide-based neoantigen vaccine [22, 23], gene therapy [24–26], immunotherapy (e.g., immune cells and checkpoint inhibitors) [2], and even nanomaterial-mediated nanotheranostics (e.g., organic nanomaterials, inorganic nanomaterials, and organic–inorganic hybrid nanomaterials). Nevertheless, the aforementioned strategies have also revealed inherent shortcomings (e.g., severe toxicity, off-target effects, graft-versus-host disease, and drug delivery barriers), which collectively hinder the further improvement in cancer administration [27, 28].

State-of-the-art renewal has highlighted the feasibility of cellular immunotherapy as promising remedy for cancer administration on the basis of the rapid progress of cryobiology and oncobiology [29–33]. For instance, pioneering and talented investigators in the field have conducted systematic and detailed studies from bench to bedside to conquer hematologic tumors and solid tumors, including the non-gene-edited natural killer (NK) cells and the CAR-transduced counterparts (e.g., CAR-T, CAR-NK cells). Distinguishing from the adaptive T cells, NK cells are adequate to efficaciously fulfill the requirement of combating the aforementioned metastatic solid tumors and hematological malignancies *via* antibody-dependent cell-mediated cytotoxicity (ADCC), direct cytolytic effect, and paracrine effects dispense with antigen presentation [2, 28, 33, 34].

Therewith, the overview of this literature aimed to summarize the current knowledge and scope of the evidence on NK cell-based immunotherapy for cancer patients from the view of cell source (e.g., peripheral blood, perinatal blood, and cell lines), *ex vivo* amplification and activation (e.g., coculture and monolayer culture), mode of action (e.g., ADCC and cytolytic effect), together with preclinical and clinical practice of NK cell-based cancer immunotherapy. Meanwhile, we also indicate the promising prospects and the concomitant challenges of NK cell-based cancer immunotherapy in regenerative medicine.

2. Natural killer (NK) cells

NK cells are pivotal part of the innate immune defense against cancer and infection, and in particular, in combating certain bacterial and viral pathogens [35]. In the

1970s, Kiessling and their colleagues firstly identified NK cells from a mouse with advantaged characteristics of cytolytic effector dispense with preliminary antigen presentation [36, 37]. Incipiently, NK cells were considered critical components to play an important role in host innate immunity and the first line of defense, and in particular, in the antiviral infection [38, 39]. To date, NK cells have been recognized as the third type of lymphocyte with vital roles in both innate and adaptive immune responses to malignancies and viral infection, which also function in delaying aging and benefiting hematopoietic reconstitution [28, 40].

As a heterogeneous lymphocyte subpopulation, NK cells can be divided into the cytotoxic $CD3^{-}CD56^{dim}CD16^{high}$ subset and the IFN-γ-producing $CD3^{-}CD56^{bright}CD16^{+}$ counterpart [28, 41]. Of note, state-of-the-art updates have also put forward the existence of long-lived memory-like NK cells with reinforced responsiveness against cancer and the CD16-dependent functional capability [42, 43].

2.1 Cell sources for NK cell generation

To date, NK cells have been generated from various origins, including umbilical cord blood (UCB) [44], placental blood [44], peripheral blood (PB)-derived mononuclear cells (PBMCs) [43, 45], NK cell lines (e.g., NK-92, YT) [28], and even derived from $CD34^{+}$ hematopoietic stem cells (HSCs) [28], human embryonic stem cells (hESCs), and induced pluripotent stem cells (iPSCs) [34, 46]. Interestingly, the content and cytotoxic activity of NK cells in perinatal and peripheral blood vary a lot. For example, NK cells take a proportion of PB cells ranging from 5–20% [47, 48], whereas the proportions of NK cells in UCB and placental blood were less than 5% [49] and 2% [50], respectively. Meanwhile, over 60% of NK cells in UCB and PB reveal the $CD3^{-}$ $CD56^{+}$ $CD16^{+}$ subset, whereas the rest belongs to the $CD3^{-}$ $CD56^{+}$ $CD16^{-}$ subset. Conversely, only 40% of NK cells in placental blood are $CD3^{-}$ $CD56^{+}$ $CD16^{+}$ cells compared with the rest $CD3^{-}CD56^{+}CD16^{-}$ subset with a percentage of 60% instead [50]. Additionally, Dogra and the colleagues found that immune responses of NK cells in diverse tissue sites were different, which indicated the tissue localization in the regulation of the NK cell development as well as the biofunctions involved in antiviral and tumor immunosurveillance [51].

During the past decades, NK cells were isolated and identified from PB to determine the specific characteristics associated with anti-infection and anticancer as well as pathogenesis (e.g., recurrent miscarriage and hematologic malignancies) [45]. PB-derived NK (PB-NK) cells have been recognized as cytotoxic innate lymphocytes, which are endowed with a unique capacity to kill a broad spectrum of virus-infected cells, cancers, and even chronic obstructive pulmonary disease (COPD) [52, 53]. Currently, PBMCs are considered the dominant ingredient for clinical- or GMP- grade NK cell manufacturing [48]. However, the stability and yield of NK cell production are far from adequate largely attributed to the limitations in blood donators and the present procedures [43, 54]. Distinguishing from those of PB-NK cells, perinatal blood-derived NK cells reveal advantaged properties such as vigorous cytolytic activity, preferable cellular vitality, and enhanced cytotoxicity [28]. Of note, the latest kinds of literature have further indicated the large-scale preparation of NK cells from human pluripotent stem cells (hPSCs), which are considered excellent candidates for "off-the-shelf" anticancer immunotherapy and NK cell development [55].

2.2 *Ex vivo* preparation of NK cells

Strategies for *ex vivo* expansion of NK cells have allowed preparing enough amounts of NK cells for clinical trials and new drug application (NDA). However, current donor cell-dependent strategies for *ex vivo* preparation of NK cells can only produce limited amount of "made-to-order" therapeutic cells for limited patients [46, 56]. For decades, a series of methods have been developed for large-scale *ex vivo* NK cell preparation, including cell sorting, feeder cell coculture (e.g., K562 cells), gene editing, low oxygen treatment, multiple cytokine cocktail stimulation, three-dimensional rotation, and bioreactors [28]. For instance, Mu *et al.* developed a simple, safe, and cost-effective strategy for *ex vivo* purification and expansion of NK cells from CB *via* zoledronate and streptococcus stimulation, and dispense of cell sorting or feeder cells/multiple cytokines within 21 days [57]. Alves *et al.* reported the *ex vivo* expansion of $CD56^+$ lymphocytes, including NK cells and NKT-like subset, from PBMCs in CellGro medium supplemented with IL-2 and fetal bovine serum (FBS), anti-CD3 (9–10 initial days) for 21 days [56]. Meanwhile, distinguishing from the resting subset, the expanded NK cells showed a higher expression level of activating receptors (e.g., CD16, NKp44, NKp46, NKG2D, NKp30, CD62L, and CD69) and a higher concentration of cytokine secretion (e.g., IFN-γ, TNF-α, and GM-CSF). Instead, Radice and the colleagues verified that PB-derived NK cells from inpatients with early-stage colorectal cancer showed enhanced *ex vivo* cytotoxicity against cancer cell lines (e.g., HT-29, K562, and human CRC Caco-2) after the stimulation of low-doses of sequential-kinetic-activated (SKA) interferon-γ (IFN-γ) *in vitro* [58].

Interestingly, we took advantage of the "3ILs"-based cell programming and induced high-efficient generation of NK cells from peripheral and perinatal blood within 14 days [43, 44]. Of note, we and other investigators in the field found that the expanded NK cells revealed elevated content and enhanced cytotoxicity against various tumor cell lines *in vitro* compared to the resident counterpart [44, 57]. Additionally, Klingemann and the colleagues tested the feasibility of a broadly applicable method for blood progenitor cell and NK cell preparation based on the well-established NK-92 cell line, which is derived from a patient with non-Hodgkin's lymphoma [59]. Collectively, NK cell expansion and activation require multiple cell signal cascades for proliferation, survival, and activation. Therewith, most of the current *ex vivo* expansion strategies are mainly focused on either using genetically modified allogeneic feeder cells or substituting the indicated factors by utilizing the autologous feeder cells [60].

2.3 Mode of action for NK cell-based cytotherapy

Aforesaid, autologous and allogeneic NK cells act as critical effector lymphocytes and mediate cancer immune clearance surveillance [61]. Generally, NK cells spontaneously function in abnormal cell elimination, pathogenic microorganism, and tumor immunosurveillance *via* ADCC, direct cytolytic effect, paracrine of cytokines, and receptor-ligand-associated natural cytotoxicity effects as well [48, 62, 63].

Generally, the mode of action for NK cell-based cytotherapy is mainly based on "NK cell education," which has also been recognized as functional maturation of NK cells. As recently reviewed by Zhang and the colleagues, this process usually involves a series of step-wise intermediate stages and obtains self-major histocompatibility complex class I (MHC-I) recognition [64]. Meanwhile, as mentioned above, the IFN-γ-producing $CD3^-CD56^{bright}$ NK cells were less mature when compared with the cytotoxic $CD3^{-}CD56^{dim}$ subset [41]. Interestingly, new insights into the long-lived memory-like NK cells indicated the enhanced CD16-dependent functional capability as well as responsiveness, which thus hold advantages over the CD25- subset in NK cell-based interventions against cancer [42, 43].

3. Chimeric antigen receptor-transduced NK (CAR-NK) cells

In recent years, CAR-transduced NK (CAR-NK) cells are considered as novel therapeutic options to reduce the incidence of relapse and recurrent cancers. A number of preclinical and clinical investigations have indicated CAR-NK cells as "off-the-shelf" products for cancer immunotherapy attributed to CAR-dependent and NK cell receptor-dependent signaling pathways [34]. Differing from those of CAR-T cells, CAR-NK cells avoid the adverse effect during cancer administration such as immune cell-associated neurotoxicity syndrome (ICANS), acute cytokine release syndrome (CRS), and graft-versus-host disease (GVHD), which thus represent the therapeutic paradigm for boosting the immune system to reinforce anticancer responses and eventually eliminate malignancies [34].

To date, a considerable number of cancer-specific antigens and the concomitant costimulatory molecules as well as the well-established subsets (e.g., NKp44, NKp46, and NKG2D) have been involved in CAR-NK cell-based immunotherapy. For example, the existing CARs transduced to generate CAR-T cells were directly transferred to NK cells, including 4-1BB, CD19, CD20, CD22, CD276, BCMA, CD3ζ, and CD28 [28, 65–70]. Simultaneously, pioneering and talented investigators in the field have dedicated themselves to optimize the constructs of CARs to enhance the efficacy of anticancer effects [32, 71]. For example, suicide genes have been integrated into the fourth generation of CARs to remove the unanticipated toxicity [72]. Furthermore, due to the advances in genome-editing techniques, the applicability and feasibility of CAR-NK cells have vastly accelerated cancer immunotherapy. Despite with deficiency in CAR constructs delivery into NK cells, a plethora of groups have highlighted the possibility for high-efficient CAR transduction *via* Lentivirus [28, 73, 74], retrovirus [75, 76], and even nonviral-mediated transfection (e.g., lipofection and electroporation, PiggyBac, and the sleeping beauty (SB) subsets) [77, 78]. Collectively, recent developments in the clinical practice of genetically modified NK cells with chimeric antigen receptors (CARs) are promising and challenging for NK cell-based immunotherapy.

4. NK cell-based cancer immunotherapy

Cancer immunotherapy with diverse preclinical and clinical attempts has been attractive and received considerable attention [79]. As time passes by, the feasibility of using NK cells in the treatment of human disorders such as refractory lung diseases, pathogenic infection, hematopoietic reconstitution, hematological malignancies, and metastatic solid tumors has increased in recent years [80]. In particular, the antileukemic potential of NK cells has raised considerable interest among researchers and clinicians for hematological malignancy administration. Nowadays, immune-based remedies characterized by the infusion of *ex vivo* activated or freshly isolated NK cells have become a research hotspot in cancer immunotherapy [34, 81–83].

In the 1980s, the dysfunction of NK cells was reported with a higher incidence of cancers, including Chédiak–Higashi syndrome and X-linked lymphoproliferative syndrome, which was first indicated in cancer immunosurveillance [41, 84, 85]. Recently, Bryce *et al.* found that NK cells in patients with chronic lymphocytic leukemia (CLL) showed reduction in content and abnormality in gene expression pattern (e.g., GATA-1, GATA-2, PU.1, and HIF-1α) in bone marrow [86].

To date, nearly 900 NK cell-based clinical trials, including the observational and interventional subtypes, were registered upon multiple tumors according to the Clinicaltrials.gov website. Generally, most of the trials were involved in hematologic malignancy administration, including acute myeloid leukemia (AML), acute lymphoblastic leukemia (ALL), chronic myelogenous leukemia (CML), and myelodysplastic syndromes (MDS). Meanwhile, clinical pieces of evidence have also indicated the therapeutic effect of NK cell-based cytotherapy upon various solid tumors such as gastric carcinoma, colorectal cancer, liver cancer, and squamous cell lung cancer [87–89]. However, the definite NK cell-based immunotherapy upon metastatic solid tumors has not been verified, which was largely attributed to the dysregulation of NK cell function and immune subversion by various factors (e.g., IDO, PGE2, and TGF-β) in the tumor microenvironment [48].

5. Discussion and conclusions

Nowadays, with the rapid progress of available remedies for cancer treatments, patients are adequate to live with the consequences of cancer. NK cells have been regarded as the first line of innate immune cells, which are involved in providing the surveillance and elimination of the stressed, infected, damaged, and malignant cells [90, 91]. NK cell-based cancer immunotherapy has largely benefited the treatments of patients for longer living and better outcomes, which also supplies new preferences for cancer administration and helps improve decisions about optimal treatment. Of note, recent kinds of literature have suggested the promising aspect of achieving considerable amount of NK cells for adoptive immunotherapy after a period of *ex vivo* expansion with multifaceted stimulation. Nevertheless, the improvement of *ex vivo* expansion procedures for the clinical application of NK cells generated under good manufacturing practice conditions is of prime importance in future.

Acknowledgements

The coauthors thank the members of Key Laboratory of Molecular Diagnostics and Precision Medicine for Surgical Oncology in Gansu Province and NHC Key Laboratory of Diagnosis and Therapy of Gastrointestinal Tumor, Gansu Provincial Hospital, Hefei Institute of Physical Science in Chinese Academy of Sciences, The First Affiliated Hospital of Shandong First Medical University, Health-Biotech (Tianjin) Stem Cell Research Institute Co., Ltd., and Jiangxi Health-Biotech Stem Cell Technology Co., Ltd. for their technical support. This work was supported by grants from the National Natural Science Foundation of China (No. 82260031), the project Youth Fund supported by Shandong Provincial Natural Science Foundation (ZR2020QC097), Fujian Provincial Ministerial Finance Special Project (2021XH018), Science and technology projects of Guizhou Province (QKH-J-ZK[2021]-107), The 2021 Central-Guided Local Science and Technology Development Fund

(ZYYDDFFZZJ-1), Medical Innovation Project of Fujian Provincial Health and Health Commission (2019-CX-21), Jiangxi Provincial Natural Science Foundation (20224BAB206077, 20212BAB216073), Key project funded by Department of Science and Technology of Shangrao City (2020AB002, 2020 K003, 2021F013), Jiangxi Provincial Key New Product Incubation Program Funded by Technical Innovation Guidance Program of Shangrao City (2020G002), the Non-profit Central Research Institute Fund of Chinese Academy of Medical Sciences (2019PT320005), and Horizontal Project upon Retrospective Analyses of COVID-19 (2020XH001).

Conflict of interest

The authors declare no conflict of interest.

Notes/thanks/other declarations

Not applicable.

Abbreviation

ADCC	Antibody-dependent cell-mediated cytotoxicity
CAR-NK	Chimeric antigen receptor-transduced NK
NK	Natural killer
PTT	Photothermal therapy
CAR-T	CAR-transduced T cells
UCB	Umbilical cord blood
PB	Peripheral blood
PBMCs	Peripheral blood-derived mononuclear cells
PB-NK	Peripheral blood-derived NK
COPD	Chronic obstructive pulmonary disease
NDA	New drug application
FBS	Fetal bovine serum
HSCs	Hematopoietic stem cells
CRS	Cytokine release syndrome
GVHD	Graft-versus-host disease
ICANS	Immune cell-associated neurotoxicity syndrome
GMP	Good manufacturing practices
CML	Chronic myelogenous leukemia
hPSCs	Human pluripotent stem cells
MDS	Myelodysplastic syndromes
ALL	Acute lymphoblastic leukemia
hESCs	Human embryonic stem cells
hiPSCs	Human induced PSCs
AML	Acute myeloid leukemia
CLL	Chronic lymphocytic leukemia
SKA	Sequential-kinetic-activated
IFN-γ	Interferon-γ

Author details

Leisheng Zhang[1,2,3,4,5]*, Xiaoming Feng[6], Zhihai Han[4] and Zhongchao Han[3,4]

1 Key Laboratory of Molecular Diagnostics and Precision Medicine for Surgical Oncology in Gansu Province and NHC Key Laboratory of Diagnosis and Therapy of Gastrointestinal Tumor, Gansu Provincial Hospital, China

2 Key Laboratory of Radiation Technology and Biophysics, Hefei Institutes of Physical Science, Chinese Academy of Sciences, China

3 Institute of Health-Biotech, Health-Biotech (Tianjin) Stem Cell Research Institute Co., Ltd., China

4 Jiangxi Research Center of Stem Cell Engineering, Jiangxi Health-Biotech Stem Cell Technology Co., Ltd., China

5 Center for Cellular Therapies, The First Affiliated Hospital of Shandong First Medical University, China

6 State Key Laboratory of Experimental Hematology, National Clinical Research Center for Blood Diseases, Haihe Laboratory of Cell Ecosystem, Institute of Hematology and Blood Diseases Hospital, Chinese Academy of Medical Sciences and Peking Union Medical College, Tianjin, China

*Address all correspondence to: leisheng_zhang@163.com

References

[1] Chen W, Zheng R, Baade PD, Zhang S, Zeng H, Bray F, et al. Cancer statistics in China, 2015. CA: a Cancer Journal for Clinicians. 2016;**66**(2):115-132

[2] Cany J, van der Waart AB, Tordoir M, Franssen GM, Hangalapura BN, de Vries J, et al. Natural killer cells generated from cord blood hematopoietic progenitor cells efficiently target bone marrow-residing human leukemia cells in NOD/SCID/IL2Rg(null) mice. PLoS One. 2013;**8**(6):e64384

[3] Qiu H, Cao S, Xu R. Cancer incidence, mortality, and burden in China: A time-trend analysis and comparison with the United States and United Kingdom based on the global epidemiological data released in. Cancer Communication, (Lond). 2020;**41**(10):1037-1048

[4] Feng RM, Zong YN, Cao SM, Xu RH. Current cancer situation in China: Good or bad news from the 2018 global cancer statistics? Cancer Communication, (Lond). 2019;**39**(1):22

[5] Wei W, Zeng H, Zheng R, Zhang S, An L, Chen R, et al. Cancer registration in China and its role in cancer prevention and control. The Lancet Oncology. 2020;**21**(7):e342-e349

[6] Sun D, Li H, Cao M, He S, Lei L, Peng J, et al. Cancer burden in China: Trends, risk factors and prevention. Cancer Biology & Medicine. 2020;**17**(4):879-895

[7] Yin P, Brauer M, Cohen AJ, Wang H, Li J, Burnett RT, et al. The effect of air pollution on deaths, disease burden, and life expectancy across China and its provinces, 1990-2017: An analysis for the global burden of disease study 2017. Lancet Planet Health. 2020;**4**(9):e386-e398

[8] Maomao C, He L, Dianqin S, Siyi H, Xinxin Y, Fan Y, et al. Current cancer burden in China: Epidemiology, etiology, and prevention. Cancer Biology & Medicine. 2022;**19**(8):1121-1138

[9] Belloni S, Arrigoni C, Caruso R. Effects from physical exercise on reduced cancer-related fatigue: A systematic review of systematic reviews and meta-analysis. Acta Oncologica. 2021;**60**(12):1678-1687

[10] Brouwers MC, Garcia K, Makarski J, Daraz L, Evidence Expert P. Team KTfCCiCPR: The landscape of knowledge translation interventions in cancer control: What do we know and where to next? A review of systematic reviews. Implementation Science. 2011;**6**:130

[11] Rowcroft A, Joh D, Pandanaboyana S, Loveday B. Hepato-pancreato-biliary and transplant surgery experience among New Zealand general surgery trainees. ANZ Journal of Surgery. 2021;**91**(6):1125-1130

[12] Ramshaw BJ. Laparoscopic surgery for cancer patients. CA: a Cancer Journal for Clinicians. 1997;**47**(6):327-350

[13] Li X, Lovell JF, Yoon J, Chen X. Clinical development and potential of photothermal and photodynamic therapies for cancer. Nature Reviews. Clinical Oncology. 2020;**17**(11):657-674

[14] Cheng L, Zhang X, Tang J, Lv Q, Liu J. Gene-engineered exosomes-thermosensitive liposomes hybrid nanovesicles by the blockade of CD47 signal for combined photothermal

therapy and cancer immunotherapy. Biomaterials. 2021;**275**:120964

[15] Kadkhoda J, Tarighatnia A, Tohidkia MR, Nader ND, Aghanejad A. Photothermal therapy-mediated autophagy in breast cancer treatment: Progress and trends. Life Sciences. 2022;**298**:120499

[16] Olivares-Urbano MA, Grinan-Lison C, Marchal JA, Nunez MI. CSC Radioresistance: A therapeutic challenge to improve radiotherapy effectiveness in cancer. Cell. 2020;**9**(7):1651

[17] Schirrmacher V. From chemotherapy to biological therapy: A review of novel concepts to reduce the side effects of systemic cancer treatment (review). International Journal of Oncology. 2019;**54**(2):407-419

[18] Kwan A, Winder N, Muthana M. Oncolytic Virotherapy treatment of breast cancer: Barriers and recent advances. Viruses. 2021;**13**(6):1128

[19] Miao L, Zhang Y, Huang L. mRNA vaccine for cancer immunotherapy. Molecular Cancer. 2021;**20**(1):41

[20] Sahin U, Oehm P, Derhovanessian E, Jabulowsky RA, Vormehr M, Gold M, et al. An RNA vaccine drives immunity in checkpoint-inhibitor-treated melanoma. Nature. 2020;**585**(7823):107-112

[21] Deli T, Orosz M, Jakab A. Hormone replacement therapy in cancer survivors - review of the literature. Pathology Oncology Research. 2020;**26**(1):63-78

[22] Ding Z, Li Q, Zhang R, Xie L, Shu Y, Gao S, et al. Personalized neoantigen pulsed dendritic cell vaccine for advanced lung cancer. Signal Transduction and Targeted Therapy. 2021;**6**(1):26

[23] Jou J, Harrington KJ, Zocca MB, Ehrnrooth E, Cohen EEW. The changing landscape of therapeutic cancer vaccines-novel platforms and Neoantigen identification. Clinical Cancer Research. 2021;**27**(3):689-703

[24] Cross D, Burmester JK. Gene therapy for cancer treatment: Past, present and future. Clinical Medicine & Research. 2006;**4**(3):218-227

[25] Graham TA, Sottoriva A. Measuring cancer evolution from the genome. The Journal of Pathology. 2017;**241**(2):183-191

[26] Lee YT, Tan YJ, Oon CE. Molecular targeted therapy: Treating cancer with specificity. European Journal of Pharmacology. 2018;**834**:188-196

[27] Mun EJ, Babiker HM, Weinberg U, Kirson ED, Von Hoff DD. Tumor-treating fields: A fourth modality in cancer treatment. Clinical Cancer Research. 2018;**24**(2):266-275

[28] Zhang L, Liu M, Yang S, Wang J, Feng X, Han Z. Natural killer cells: Of-the-shelf cytotherapy for cancer immunosurveillance. American Journal of Cancer Research. 2021;**11**(4):1770-1791

[29] Depil S, Duchateau P, Grupp SA, Mufti G, Poirot L. 'Off-the-shelf' allogeneic CAR T cells: Development and challenges. Nature Reviews. Drug Discovery. 2020;**19**(3):185-199

[30] Hernandez-Lopez A, Tellez-Gonzalez MA, Mondragon-Teran P, Meneses-Acosta A. Chimeric antigen receptor-T cells: A pharmaceutical scope. Frontiers in Pharmacology. 2021;**12**:720692

[31] Liu E, Marin D, Banerjee P, Macapinlac HA, Thompson P, Basar R,

et al. Use of CAR-transduced natural killer cells in CD19-positive lymphoid tumors. The New England Journal of Medicine. 2020;**382**(6):545-553

[32] Siegler EL, Zhu Y, Wang P, Yang L. Off-the-shelf CAR-NK cells for cancer immunotherapy. Cell Stem Cell. 2018;**23**(2):160-161

[33] Wrona E, Borowiec M, Potemski P. CAR-NK cells in the treatment of solid tumors. International Journal of Molecular Sciences. 2021;**22**(11):5899

[34] Zhang L, Meng Y, Feng X, Han Z. CAR-NK cells for cancer immunotherapy: From bench to bedside. Biomarker Research. 2022;**10**(1):12

[35] Orange JS. Natural killer cell deficiency. The Journal of Allergy and Clinical Immunology. 2013;**132**(3):515-525

[36] Kiessling R, Klein E, Wigzell H. "natural" killer cells in the mouse. I. Cytotoxic cells with specificity for mouse Moloney leukemia cells. Specificity and distribution according to genotype. European Journal of Immunology. 1975;**5**(2):112-117

[37] Kiessling R, Klein E, Pross H, Wigzell H. "natural" killer cells in the mouse. II. Cytotoxic cells with specificity for mouse Moloney leukemia cells. Characteristics of the killer cell. European Journal of Immunology. 1975;**5**(2):117-121

[38] Wu F, Xie M, Hun M, She Z, Li C, Luo S, et al. Natural killer cell-derived extracellular vesicles: Novel players in cancer immunotherapy. Frontiers in Immunology. 2021;**12**:658698

[39] Mancini M, Vidal SM. Mechanisms of natural killer cell evasion through viral adaptation. Annual Review of Immunology. 2020;**38**:511-539

[40] O'Brien KL, Finlay DK. Immunometabolism and natural killer cell responses. Nature Reviews. Immunology. 2019;**19**(5):282-290

[41] Morvan MG, Lanier LL. NK cells and cancer: You can teach innate cells new tricks. Nature Reviews. Cancer. 2016;**16**(1):7-19

[42] Capuano C, Battella S, Pighi C, Franchitti L, Turriziani O, Morrone S, et al. Tumor-targeting anti-CD20 antibodies mediate In vitro expansion of memory natural killer cells: Impact of CD16 affinity ligation conditions and In vivo priming. Frontiers in Immunology. 2018;**9**:1031

[43] Liu M, Meng Y, Zhang L, Han Z, Feng X. High-efficient generation of natural killer cells from peripheral blood with preferable cell vitality and enhanced cytotoxicity by combination of IL-2, IL-15 and IL-18. Biochemical and Biophysical Research Communications. 2021;**534**:149-156

[44] Zhang L, Liu M, Song B, Miao W, Zhan R, Yang S, et al. Decoding the multidimensional signatures of resident and expanded natural killer cells generated from perinatal blood. American Journal of Cancer Research. 2022;**12**(5):2132-2145

[45] Guerrero B, Hassouneh F, Delgado E, Casado JG, Tarazona R. Natural killer cells in recurrent miscarriage: An overview. Journal of Reproductive Immunology. 2020;**142**:103209

[46] Zeng J, Tang SY, Toh LL, Wang S. Generation of "off-the-shelf" natural killer cells from peripheral blood cell-derived induced pluripotent stem cells. Stem Cell Reports. 2017;**9**(6):1796-1812

[47] Koepsell SA, Miller JS, McKenna DH Jr. Natural killer cells: A review

of manufacturing and clinical utility. Transfusion. 2013;**53**(2):404-410

[48] Guillerey C, Huntington ND, Smyth MJ. Targeting natural killer cells in cancer immunotherapy. Nature Immunology. 2016;**17**(9):1025-1036

[49] Balassa K, Rocha V. Anticancer cellular immunotherapies derived from umbilical cord blood. Expert Opinion on Biological Therapy. 2018;**18**(2):121-134

[50] Kang L, Voskinarian-Berse V, Law E, Reddin T, Bhatia M, Hariri A, et al. Characterization and ex vivo expansion of human placenta-derived natural killer cells for cancer immunotherapy. Frontiers in Immunology. 2013;**4**:101

[51] Dogra P, Rancan C, Ma W, Toth M, Senda T, Carpenter DJ, et al. Tissue determinants of human NK cell development, function, and residence. Cell. 2020;**180**(4):749-763 e713

[52] Kim JM, Yi E, Cho H, Choi WS, Ko DH, Yoon DH, et al. Assessment of NK cell activity based on NK cell-specific receptor synergy in peripheral blood mononuclear cells and whole blood. International Journal of Molecular Sciences. 2020;**21**(21):8112

[53] Rao Y, Le Y, Xiong J, Pei Y, Sun Y. NK cells in the pathogenesis of chronic obstructive pulmonary disease. Frontiers in Immunology. 2021;**12**:666045

[54] Blum KS, Pabst R. Lymphocyte numbers and subsets in the human blood. Do they mirror the situation in all organs? Immunology Letters. 2007;**108**(1):45-51

[55] Li Y, Hermanson DL, Moriarity BS, Kaufman DS. Human iPSC-derived natural killer cells engineered with chimeric antigen receptors enhance anti-tumor activity. Cell Stem Cell. 2018;**23**(2):181-192 e185

[56] Alves PCM, De Angelo Andrade LAL, Petta CA, Lorand-Metze I, Derchain SF, Guimaraes F. Ex vivo expansion of CD56+ NK and NKT-like lymphocytes from peripheral blood mononuclear cells of patients with ovarian neoplasia. Scandinavian Journal of Immunology. 2011;**74**(3):244-252

[57] Mu YX, Zhao YX, Li BY, Bao HJ, Jiang H, Qi XL, et al. A simple method for in vitro preparation of natural killer cells from cord blood. BMC Biotechnology. 2019;**19**(1):80

[58] Radice E, Miranda V, Bellone G. Low-doses of sequential-kinetic-activated interferon-gamma enhance the ex vivo cytotoxicity of peripheral blood natural killer cells from patients with early-stage colorectal cancer. A preliminary study. Int Immunopharmacol. 2014;**19**(1):66-73

[59] Klingemann HG, Wong E, Maki G. A cytotoxic NK-cell line (NK-92) for ex vivo purging of leukemia from blood. Biology of Blood and Marrow Transplantation. 1996;**2**(2):68-75

[60] Becker PS, Suck G, Nowakowska P, Ullrich E, Seifried E, Bader P, et al. Selection and expansion of natural killer cells for NK cell-based immunotherapy. Cancer Immunology, Immunotherapy. 2016;**65**(4):477-484

[61] Woan KV, Miller JS. Harnessing natural killer cell antitumor immunity: From the bench to bedside. Cancer Immunology Research. 2019;**7**(11):1742-1747

[62] Freud AG, Mundy-Bosse BL, Yu J, Caligiuri MA. The broad Spectrum of human natural killer cell diversity. Immunity. 2017;**47**(5):820-833

[63] Hodgins JJ, Khan ST, Park MM, Auer RC, Ardolino M. Killers 2.0: NK cell therapies at the forefront of cancer control. The Journal of Clinical Investigation. 2019;**129**(9):3499-3510

[64] Vivier E. What is natural in natural killer cells? Immunology Letters. 2006;**107**(1):1-7

[65] Jayaraman J, Mellody MP, Hou AJ, Desai RP, Fung AW, Pham AHT, et al. CAR-T design: Elements and their synergistic function. eBioMedicine. 2020;**58**:102931

[66] Zhang Y, Li Y, Cao W, Wang F, Xie X, Li Y, et al. Single-cell analysis of target antigens of CAR-T reveals a potential landscape of "on-target, off-tumor toxicity". Frontiers in Immunology. 2021;**12**:799206

[67] Genssler S, Burger MC, Zhang C, Oelsner S, Mildenberger I, Wagner M, et al. Dual targeting of glioblastoma with chimeric antigen receptor-engineered natural killer cells overcomes heterogeneity of target antigen expression and enhances antitumor activity and survival. Oncoimmunology. 2016;**5**(4):e1119354

[68] Imai C, Iwamoto S, Campana D. Genetic modification of primary natural killer cells overcomes inhibitory signals and induces specific killing of leukemic cells. Blood. 2005;**106**(1):376-383

[69] Xu Y, Liu Q, Zhong M, Wang Z, Chen Z, Zhang Y, et al. 2B4 costimulatory domain enhancing cytotoxic ability of anti-CD5 chimeric antigen receptor engineered natural killer cells against T cell malignancies. Journal of Hematology & Oncology. 2019;**12**(1):49

[70] Romanski A, Uherek C, Bug G, Seifried E, Klingemann H, Wels WS, et al. CD19-CAR engineered NK-92 cells are sufficient to overcome NK cell resistance in B-cell malignancies. Journal of Cellular and Molecular Medicine. 2016;**20**(7):1287-1294

[71] Sanmamed MF, Chen L. A paradigm shift in cancer immunotherapy: From enhancement to normalization. Cell. 2018;**175**(2):313-326

[72] Daher M, Rezvani K. Outlook for new CAR-based therapies with a focus on CAR NK cells: What lies beyond CAR-engineered T cells in the race against cancer. Cancer Discovery. 2021;**11**(1):45-58

[73] Oelsner S, Friede ME, Zhang C, Wagner J, Badura S, Bader P, et al. Continuously expanding CAR NK-92 cells display selective cytotoxicity against B-cell leukemia and lymphoma. Cytotherapy. 2017;**19**(2):235-249

[74] Boissel L, Betancur-Boissel M, Lu W, Krause DS, Van Etten RA, Wels WS, et al. Retargeting NK-92 cells by means of CD19- and CD20-specific chimeric antigen receptors compares favorably with antibody-dependent cellular cytotoxicity. Oncoimmunology. 2013;**2**(10):e26527

[75] Imamura M, Shook D, Kamiya T, Shimasaki N, Chai SM, Coustan-Smith E, et al. Autonomous growth and increased cytotoxicity of natural killer cells expressing membrane-bound interleukin-15. Blood. 2014;**124**(7):1081-1088

[76] Guven H, Konstantinidis KV, Alici E, Aints A, Abedi-Valugerdi M, Christensson B, et al. Efficient gene transfer into primary human natural killer cells by retroviral transduction. Experimental Hematology. 2005;**33**(11):1320-1328

[77] Rostovskaya M, Fu J, Obst M, Baer I, Weidlich S, Wang H, et al.

Transposon-mediated BAC transgenesis in human ES cells. Nucleic Acids Research. 2012;**40**(19):e150

[78] Vargas JE, Chicaybam L, Stein RT, Tanuri A, Delgado-Canedo A, Bonamino MH. Retroviral vectors and transposons for stable gene therapy: Advances, current challenges and perspectives. Journal of Translational Medicine. 2016;**14**(1):288

[79] Yang YJ, Park JC, Kim HK, Kang JH, Park SY. A trial of autologous ex vivo-expanded NK cell-enriched lymphocytes with docetaxel in patients with advanced non-small cell lung cancer as second- or third-line treatment: Phase IIa study. Anticancer Research. 2013;**33**(5):2115-2122

[80] Guimaraes F, Guven H, Donati D, Christensson B, Ljunggren HG, Bejarano MT, et al. Evaluation of ex vivo expanded human NK cells on antileukemia activity in SCID-beige mice. Leukemia. 2006;**20**(5):833-839

[81] Yu SJ, Ma C, Heinrich B, Brown ZJ, Sandhu M, Zhang Q, et al. Targeting the crosstalk between cytokine-induced killer cells and myeloid-derived suppressor cells in hepatocellular carcinoma. Journal of Hepatology. 2019;**70**(3):449-457

[82] Zhang C, Burger MC, Jennewein L, Genßler S, Schönfeld K, Zeiner P, et al. ErbB2/HER2-specific NK cells for targeted therapy of glioblastoma. Journal of the National Cancer Institute. 6 Dec 2015;**108**(5)

[83] Zhang Q, Zhang H, Ding J, Liu H, Li H, Li H, et al. Combination therapy with EpCAM-CAR-NK-92 cells and Regorafenib against human colorectal cancer models. Journal of Immunology Research. 2018;**2018**:4263520

[84] Roder JC, Haliotis T, Klein M, Korec S, Jett JR, Ortaldo J, et al. A new immunodeficiency disorder in humans involving NK cells. Nature. 1980;**284**(5756):553-555

[85] Sullivan JL, Byron KS, Brewster FE, Purtilo DT. Deficient natural killer cell activity in x-linked lymphoproliferative syndrome. Science. 1980;**210**(4469):543-545

[86] Manso BA, Zhang H, Mikkelson MG, Gwin KA, Secreto CR, Ding W, et al. Bone marrow hematopoietic dysfunction in untreated chronic lymphocytic leukemia patients. Leukemia. 2019;**33**(3):638-652

[87] Ishigami S, Natsugoe S, Tokuda K, Nakajo A, Xiangming C, Iwashige H, et al. Clinical impact of intratumoral natural killer cell and dendritic cell infiltration in gastric cancer. Cancer Letters. 2000;**159**(1):103-108

[88] Villegas FR, Coca S, Villarrubia VG, Jimenez R, Chillon MJ, Jareno J, et al. Prognostic significance of tumor infiltrating natural killer cells subset CD57 in patients with squamous cell lung cancer. Lung Cancer. 2002;**35**(1):23-28

[89] Zheng X, Qian Y, Fu B, Jiao D, Jiang Y, Chen P, et al. Mitochondrial fragmentation limits NK cell-based tumor immunosurveillance. Nature Immunology. 2019;**20**(12):1656-1667

[90] Huang RS, Lai MC, Lin S. Ex vivo expansion and CRISPR-Cas9 genome editing of primary human natural killer cells. Current Protocols. 2021;**1**(9):e246

[91] Heipertz EL, Zynda ER, Stav-Noraas TE, Hungler AD, Boucher SE, Kaur N, et al. Current perspectives on "off-the-shelf" allogeneic NK and CAR-NK cell therapies. Frontiers in Immunology. 2021;**12**:732135

Section 2

Natural Killer Cells for Cancer Immunotherapy

Chapter 2

Natural Killer Cell-Based Cancer Immunotherapy: From Bench to Bedside

Li Zhang and Chang Liu

Abstract

Natural killer (NK) cells are innate cytotoxic lymphocytes involved in the surveillance and elimination of cancer. The increasing number of studies have identified novel methods for enhancing the anti-tumor immunity of NK cells and expanding NK cells *ex vivo*, which paved the way for a new generation of anticancer immunotherapies. In this chapter, we will review the following aspects regarding NK cells, including the inhibitory and activating receptors modulating NK cell activity, NK cell development, the cytotoxic mechanism of NK cells, isolation, expansion and characterization of NK cells, and the source for NK cells. Moreover, we will highlight the cutting-edge immunotherapeutic strategies in preclinical and clinical development such as chimeric antigen receptor (CAR)-NK cells, as well as the adoptive NK transfer to target cancer stem cells (CSCs). Last, we will discuss the challenges NK cells face which should be overcome to achieve cancer clearance.

Keywords: natural killer (NK) cells, expansion, cancer immunotherapy, cancer stem cell (CSC), CAR-NK

1. Introduction

Activating the immune system by immunotherapy is an innovative way to target cancers. Immune checkpoints such as cytotoxic T lymphocyte antigen-4 (CTLA-4), programmed death-1 (PD-1), lymphocyte activation gene-3 (LAG-3), T cell immunoglobulin, and ITIM domain (TIGIT) are the most studied ones. PD-1 and CLTA-4 have received great attention since the blockage of PD-1 or CTLA-4 signaling improved the tumor patient survival significantly. Immune checkpoints consist of pairs of receptors-ligands present in immune cells as well as tumor cells, and the interaction of the receptors in tumor cells with their ligands in immune cells inhibits the immune activity of immune cells. Immune checkpoint blockade has been regarded as the recovery of cytotoxic lymphocyte activity. However, partial or complete loss of HLA-I expression has been attributed to be one of the immune escape mechanisms in tumors, which evade T-cell surveillance [1]. Under these circumstances, the cytotoxic T cells and NK cells, which are capable of recognizing and killing tumor cells despite of HLA-I expression, seem to be vital [2–4]. Immune checkpoints have been mainly studied in T cells, but NK cells are also affected by these interactions.

NK cells, which are cytotoxic lymphocytes with high antitumor, antiviral, and antimicrobial activities in the innate immune system, were first identified as lymphoid subsets and were critical mediators of antitumor immunity [5]. NK cells were capable of responding to a variety of infections as well as transformed cells by directly killing and secreting pro-inflammation cytokines without prior antigen sensitization or recognition of specific tumor antigens [6, 7]. NK cells develop at numerous sites including bone marrow, lymph nodes, secondary lymphoid organs, thymus, liver, gut, and tonsils [8], and the effector functions are similar to $CD8^+$ T cells. $CD56^{dim}$ and $CD56^{bright}$ cells are the two subsets of human NK cells, which have distinct immune phenotypes and functions. In peripheral blood, $CD56^{dim}$ cells constitute 90% of NK cells, and they have strong cytotoxic capability, while $CD56^{bright}$ subset is mostly involved in cytokine production. The NK cells in the secondary lymphoid tissue are different from the NK cells in the peripheral blood.

There have been many efforts to exploit these potent effector cells such as NK cells or T cells either by endogenous activation or by adoptive transfer. Unlike donor T cells, NK cells do not induce graft-versus-host disease (GVHD). It would be highly likely that NK cells would exploit an important position targeting tumors with deficient HLA-I molecules.

2. NK cell regulation and NK cell-based cancer immunotherapy

2.1 NK cell activity regulation

It was hypothesized that NK cells were derived from $CD34^+CD45RA^+$ hematopoietic progenitor cells (HSC). NK precursors were identified in the hematopoietic population and differentiated into NK cells. Several transcription factors such as Ets-1, Id2, Ikaros, and PU as well as soluble and membrane factors were involved in the regulation of the NK cell phenotypic and functional maturation [9–11]. Moreover, IL-15-dependent signaling pathway plays an essential role in NK cell development, homeostasis, and survival.

In healthy individuals, 90% of NK cells in peripheral blood are mature with $CD16^{bright}$ and $CD56^{dim}$ expression. The rest of the NK cells are an immature subset, which is $CD16^{dim}$ or $CD16^-$, $CD56^{bright}$, and $CD25^+$, and the main function of these NK cells is to produce cytokines [12].

It was found that lymphoma cells that lost MHC class I surface molecules could be killed by NK cells, but the original MHC class I^+ cells were otherwise resistant. This phenomenon drives the hypothesis that NK cells are able to sense the absence of "self" MHC class-I molecules on target cells [13]. Years later, the hypothesis was verified by the discovery of inhibitory as well as activating NK receptors.

NK cell activity is modulated and controlled by a series of inhibitory and activating NK cell receptors. The inhibitory receptors in humans are mainly inhibitory killer Ig-like receptors (KIRs). KIRs consist of long cytoplasmic tails containing two ITIM domains, recruiting tyrosine phosphatases to transduce inhibitory signals, followed by two (KIR2D) or three (KIR3D) polymorphic extracellular Ig-like domains. The inhibitory KIRs recognize and directly interact with the human leukocyte antigen (HLA) class-I alleles and CD94/NKG2A heterodimer, especially the non-classical HLA-E molecule [14–16]. Different HLA class I allotypes contained the same specific epitopes, which are recognized by distinct KIRs. However, when a KIR-HLA-I mismatch or the loss of HLA-I occurs, inhibitory KIRs cannot interact with their ligands to activate NK cells [17].

The activating NK cell receptors play a fundamental role in the recognition and killing of transformed or virus-infected cells, which have normal HLA-I molecule expression, through direct interaction with ligands expressed [18–20]. These activating receptors contain the following families: activating KIRs, C-type lectin-like receptors, natural cytotoxicity receptors (NCR), and signaling lymphocyte activating molecule (SLAM) family of receptors [21].

A large number of activating NK cell receptors is responsible for the existence of 6000-30,000 different phenotypic NK populations, providing flexibility to respond to pathogens and tumor cells [22]. CD94/NKG2A in the C-type lectin-like receptor family was the first HLA-I-specific receptor expressed by the most immature $CD56^{bright}$ cells during NK cell differentiation. After a few steps of maturation, $CD56^{dim}$ NK cells replace the $CD56^{bright}$ cells; in addition, $CD56^{dim}$ NK cells carry KIR receptors but abandon NKG2A [23–25]. So most mature NK cells express KIR as well as the terminal differentiation marker CD57 [26]. HLA-I-specific inhibitory receptors normally prevent auto-reactive responses by the recognition of autologous cells. Nevertheless, for tumors, HLA-I-specific inhibitory receptors function as immune checkpoints to restrain the cytotoxic activity of NK cells [3, 27]. PD-1, a non-HLA-I specific inhibitory receptor, might be also expressed in NK cells. PD-1 was originally discovered in T cells and played a sharp inhibitory role in their tumor-killing activity. PD-1 is expressed on mature NK cells, which are $KIR^{+}CD57^{+}NKG2A^{-}$ cells, under normal conditions. However, for patients with tumors, the proportions of $PD\text{-}1^{+}$ NK cells were increased significantly [28, 29]. Some other immune checkpoints are also expressed by NK cells to recognize additional ligands, including CTLA-4, T cell immunoglobulin and mucin-domain-containing molecule 3 (TIM-3), lymphocyte activation gene 3 (LAG-3), T cell immune receptor with Ig and immune receptor tyrosine-based inhibition motif domains (TIGIT), and CD96 [4, 30, 31].

The inhibitory receptors recognize self-MHC class I molecule to inhibit NK cell activation, which enables the self-tolerance and prevents host cell killing. NK cells will be activated when they encounter the cells that are lack of MHC class I molecule, which is known as the "missing-self" hypothesis [32]. Through the recognition of MHC class I molecules, NK cells distinguish transformed or infected cells from normal host cells, and these abnormal cells with a lack of MHC class I expression or high expression of "stress ligands" could be lysed by NK cells. MHC class I molecules were usually downregulated in the tumor cells to escape the immune surveillance of cytotoxic T lymphocytes. Nevertheless, NK cells would still be activated and attack these tumor cells, since the activation receptors are no longer suppressed under these circumstances to induce potent stimulatory signals [33, 34].

2.2 NK cell development

NK cell development occurs predominantly within the bone marrow. At first, NK cell is referred to as a common lymphoid progenitor (CLP), which is identified by some markers including stem cells antigen-1 (Sca-1), c-kit (CD117), interleukin-7 receptor (IL-7Ra), and FMS-like tyrosine kinase-3 (Flt-3). Then, the CLP develops into a pre-NK precursor (pre-NKP) consisting of NK precursors and innate lymphoid cell precursors. Next, the pre-NKP becomes NKP and expresses IL-15 receptor complex (IL-15Rβ/γ) to maintain long-term NK cell development and survival. During this stage, symbolic NK cell marker CD56 is expressed, and NK cells are further subdivided into the immature $CD56^{bright}$ subset and mature $CD56^{dim}$ subset. $CD56^{bright}$ NK cells participated in immunomodulation through secreting cytokine

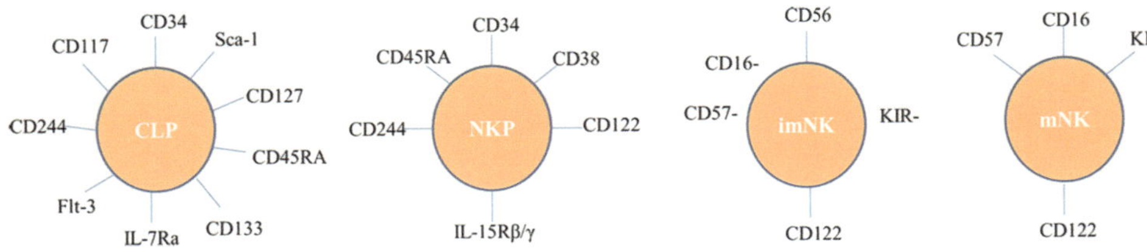

Figure 1.
The specific markers expression on CLP, NKP, immature NK (imNK) cells, and mature NK (mNK) cells during NK cell development.

interferon-gamma (IFNγ). While CD56dim NK cells which are the dominant cells in the peripheral blood and spleen have cytotoxic ability (**Figure 1**).

During immune response, NK cells can receive signals from other immune cells as well as tumor cells. For example, dendritic cells regulate the proliferation and immune function development of NK cells through the secretion of IL-12, type I IFN, trans-presenting IL-15, and secretory exosomes [35, 36]. And $CD4^+$ cells could regulate NK cell proliferation and survival by IL-2. On the contrary, the regulatory T (Treg) cells can suppress NK cell proliferation and function through transforming growth factor beta (TGF-β) [37, 38].

2.3 The cytotoxic mechanism of NK cells

The death receptor pathway and the granule-dependent pathway are classic NK cell cytotoxic mechanisms. The two predominant pathways jointly induce the apoptosis of the target cells. The former one is a caspase-dependent apoptosis pathway, activated by the tumor necrosis factor (e.g., Fas/CD95) on target cells with their equivalent ligands such as FasL and tumor necrosis factor-related apoptosis-inducing ligand (TRAIL) on NK cells [23, 39]. TRAIL and FASL interact with their receptors on the targeting cells. Interaction between FASL and FAS as well as TRAIL and TRAIL receptors promotes death-inducing signaling complex formation, which includes Fas-associated death domain protein (FADD), caspase-8, along with caspase-10 [40]. Caspase-8 activation leads to the activation of the other caspases or Bid proteolysis, resulting in the subsequent caspase activation as well as cytochrome C release [23].

After identifying and bounding to the target cells, NK cells initiate the granule-dependent pathway to deliver the granzymes, which are cytotoxic granules containing perforin and proteases to kill the target cells [41]. Distinct granzymes (A, B, H, K, and M) activate different apoptotic or non-apoptotic cell death pathways. Granzyme A activates non-apoptotic cell death, and Granzyme B activates apoptosis by activating caspases as well as by cytochrome C release. Granzymes H, K, and M were less studied, and it was reported that $CD56^{bright}$ cells released Granzymes K to mediate the non-apoptotic tumor cell death [42]. Granzyme H was shown to help remove infected and transformed cells. And Granzyme M functioned as an anti-tumor effector after adoptive NK cell transfer [43]. The death receptor pathway and the granule-dependent pathway endow NK cells with the different killing abilities to eliminate different tumor cells.

B7-H3 was reported to be correlated with the poor prognosis of cancer patients, through the inhibition of NK cell activity; on the contrary, the inhibition of B7-H3 restrains tumor growth and increases the cytotoxic activity of NK cells [44]. Moreover, the tumor cells can also be killed by antibody-dependent cellular cytotoxicity (ADCC), as they express a low-affinity Fc receptor for IgG, FcεRIII.

2.4 NK cell isolation, expansion, and characterization

The commercial NK isolation kits were available nowadays. The commonly used peripheral blood NK cell isolation kit was Miltenyi Biotec. NK cells could be either isolated from peripheral blood directly as well as from the peripheral blood mononuclear cells (PBMCs). In this regard, PBMCs should be isolated from the peripheral blood first. Layer 35 mL of peripheral blood on 15 mL of Ficoll-Paque, and then centrifuge at 400 g for 20 minutes without brake. Harvest the PBMCs from the interface of Ficoll-Paque and plasma, and wash the three times with PBS (centrifuge at 400g for 10 minutes). NK cell isolation protocol is as follows: Pass PBMCs through a 30-μm filter to remove cell clump, and then centrifuge cell suspension at 500 g for 7 minutes to count cells. Use precooled solutions to keep cells cold, resuspend 10^7 cells in 40 μl solution, and add 10 μl of biotin-conjugated antibodies cocktail to remove unwanted cells. Then, add 30 μl of separation buffer and 20 μl of MicroBeads, mix well, and incubate for 10 min at 4 °C. Wash once in separation buffer (centrifuge at 500 g for 7 minutes) and resuspend labeled cells in 500-μl separation buffer. Place an MS column in the magnetic field of the MACS separator and pre-rinse with separation buffer. Apply cell suspension to the column. Collect the flow-through fraction containing enriched untouched NK cells. Wash the column three times with separation buffer, and also collect the NK cells.

As to isolate the NK cells from the peripheral blood instead of PBMCs, use the RosetteSep™ Human NK Cell Enrichment Cocktail from STEM CELL Technologies. Transfer 10 ml whole blood in a 50-mL tube, and add 500 μl RosetteSep Human NK Cell Enrichment Cocktail, incubate for 20 min at room temperature and mix gently. Dilute the sample with RPMI with 2% FBS (1:1), mix gently, and lay on Lympholyte-H cell separation media. Centrifuge for 20 min at room temperature at 800 g without brake. Collect enriched NK cells from the interface of Lympholyte-H and plasma, and wash the NK cells twice with a complete medium. Either way, NK cell number and viability should be determined by Trypan Blue dye exclusion, in addition to assess NK cell purity by flow cytometry.

NK cell expansion requires multiple signals for survival, activation, and proliferation. In the early years, *in vivo* expand NK cells were the main purpose of the clinical trials. Administrating systemic cytokines, mainly IL-2, did not improve the clinical outcome of cancer patients due to the serious side effects of cytokines [45]. Additionally, IL-2 also stimulates the regulatory T cell, which plays the immunosuppression effect. Thus, *ex vivo* NK cell stimulation with other cytokines can also help to increase the survivability of the NK cells. NK cell expansion can be initiated from both PBMCs and purified NK cells using the following protocol. The initiating number of PBMCs or NK cells can be varied based on the amount of NK cells desired after expansion. For each $5{\times}10^6$ cell to be expanded, count and irradiate 10^7 K562 Cl9 mIL21 using a gamma irradiator at 100 Gy. Wash the K562 cells with PBS and resuspend in NK cell expansion media (NKEM) after the irradiation. Seed $5{\times}10^6$ PBMCs with 10^7 irradiated K562 Cl9 mIL21 in 40 mL of NKEM in a T75 flask and place it upright in an incubator at 37°C and 5% CO_2. After 5 days, collect NK cells by centrifugation and replace half of the media with fresh NKEM. Count the number of cells after a week. For every $5{\times}10^6$ cell, count and irradiate $5{\times}10^6$ K562 Cl9 mIL21 as previously described. Add an equal number of irradiated K562 Cl9 mIL21 and resuspend in NKEM with the density of $2.5{\times}10^5$ cells/ml, then seed cells in T75 flasks. After 10 days, change the entire media with fresh NKEM based on the cell numbers. Resuspend NK cells with the irradiated same amount of K562 Cl9 mIL21 in NKEM and change the whole media with fresh NKEM after 17 days. At the end of the expansion, count the cell number and analyze the NK cell phenotyping.

It was reported that *in vitro* pre-activation of NK cells with novel cytokines such as IL-12, IL-15, and IL-18 induces CD25 expression in NK cells [46]. Thus, expansion strategies have been focused either to substitute these factors using autologous feeder cells or to use genetically modified allogeneic feeder cells. Autologous PBMC as feeder cells to expand NK cells *in vitro* has been shown to generate enough functional active NK cells [47]. The number of purified NK cells increased 2500 folds after 17 days by using autologous PBMCs as feeder cells. Combined feeder cells with OKT3 and IL-2 endowed NK cells with cytolytic activity against tumor cells [48]. Genetically modified K562 cells or Epstein-Barr virus-transformed lymphoblastoid cell lines were used as feeder cells for NK cell expansion. The leukemia cell line K562 was genetically altered to express a membrane-bound form of IL-15 and the 4-1BB (CD137L) [49]. By using this feeder cell, NK cells were expanded by 277-fold after 3 weeks [49]. K562 feeder cells expressing CD137L, MICA, and soluble IL-15 were also produced, and they promoted the NK cell expansion of 550 folds [50]. Denman et al. have constructed K562-based feeder cells with the expression of membrane-bound chimeras of IL-21 (mbIL21) and IL-15 (mbIL15), and investigated NK cell expansion, phenotype, and function. It was found that IL-21 was superior to IL-15 in terms of promoting NK cell growth, but as to NK phenotype or function, the function of IL-21 and IL-15 expressing k562 feeder cells had no significant differences [51].

NK cells are characterized by a lack of CD3/TCR molecules and expression of CD16 and CD56 surface antigens. $CD56^{dim}$ NK cells express high levels of CD16, while $CD56^{bright}$ NK cells are $CD16^{dim}$ or negative [52]. Cytotoxicity of NK cells against various malignant cell lines, and the expression patterns of NK cell receptors including cluster of differentiation (CD)-16, CD69, CD158b, natural killer group-2 member D (NKG2D), NKp30, NKp44, NKp46 define NK cell activity [53]. The cytotoxic assay of NK cells was performed as follows, using $6{\times}10^5$ NK cells and $3{\times}10^5$ target cells to perform the experiment. Resuspend 10^6 target cells in 1 ml of NKEM composed of Calcein-AM, incubated for 1 hour at 37 °C, with occasional shaking. Prepare NK cells at $1{\times}10^6$ cells/ ml, add 200 ul of NK cell suspension to 3 wells of a 96-well plate corresponding To 10:1 (E:T) ratio. Dilute the NK cells for the five subsequent E:T ratios. After 1 hour of calcein loading, wash target cells in NKEM twice, centrifuging for 5 minutes at 1200 rpm. Re-count the target cells and resuspend at $1{\times}10^5$ cells/ml. Add 10^4 target cells to NK cells, and centrifuge for 1 minute at 100 g to enable cell contact. Then, incubate the cell mixture at 37 °C and 5% CO2 for 4 hours. Mix them gently, centrifuge at 100g for 5 minutes to pellet the cells, and transfer 100 μl of the supernatant to a new plate. Read the absorbance (excitation filter 485 nm, emission filter 530 nm). Calculate Percent Specific Lysis according to the formula [(test release-spontaneous release)/(maximum release - spontaneous release)] × 100 [54].

2.5 Source of NK cells

It was agreed that NK cell transfer is safe and well-tolerated by patients. Interleukin (IL) 2 was administered to activate NK cells *in vitro* or *in vivo* after immunosuppressive treatment by fludarabine and cyclophosphamide.

Nevertheless, adoptive transfer of NK cells for cancer immunotherapy has been hindered by the inability to obtain sufficient NK cells, as these cells represent a small fraction (about 10% comprise the third largest population of lymphocytes following

B and T cells) of blood mononuclear cells, and long-term expansion and persistence of NK cells *ex vivo* was still a challenge. Moreover, the alloreactive T cells would eliminate NK cells after transfer [55, 56].

Various protocols have been used to isolate and preferentially expand primary NK cells from PBMC [57]. The combination of cell selection and depletion using immunomagnetic beads was the common protocol [58]. Leukapheresis products were used for the clinical-grade purification of NK cells by depleting CD3$^+$ cells followed by the selection of CD56$^+$ cells [59] or in combination with subsequent a 14-day of stimulation with IL-2 [60]. It was reported that autologous adoptive NK-cell therapy had drawbacks, which were mainly that self-MHC I molecules on the tumor cells inhibited NK cells. So the autologous adoptive transfer of NK cells may not be efficient, and healthy allogeneic NK cells were an optimal option.

Since a large number of activating and inhibitory receptors, cooperative receptor pairs, and overlapping signaling pathways involved in NK cell maturation, activation, and proliferation, it is difficult to identify signaling molecules to expand NK cells *in vitro* [61]. NK cell propagation *in vitro* needs feeder cells [62], various cytokines such as IL-2, IL-15, IL-21 [63, 64], as well as fusion proteins [65, 66].

In umbilical cord blood, NK cells account for about 30% of lymphocytes. In contrast, NK cells account for 10% of lymphocytes in peripheral blood. Furthermore, the immunophenotype of NK cells from umbilical cord blood is CD3-CD56$^+$, which is roughly classified as the less differentiated CD56bright and mature CD56dim NK cells in a broad sense. CD34$^+$ hematopoietic progenitors from umbilical cord blood or bone marrow are considered as an excellent source for cell therapeutic applications [67]. Previously, it was a challenge to obtain efficient numbers of NK cells for the low number of NK cells in cord blood. In recent years, different protocols have been developed for the generation of NK cells from CD34+ cells from bone marrow as well as cord blood through co-cultured with stromal cell lines and a combination of cytokines [68–70]. More recently, *ex vivo* expansion protocol of NK cells, derived from cord blood CD34+ cells, has been established. This method uses a clinical-grade serum-free culture medium and a mixture of cytokines as a substitute for the extracellular microenvironment of bone marrow in static cell culture bags and an automated bioreactor without feeder cells [71]. Up to 10^{10} NK cells derived from CD34+ cells were possible by adding high levels of several activating receptors such as NKG2D and NC [72].

The healthy allogeneic NK cells can be sourced from UCB, adult donor lymphopoiesis products, or even from NK-cell lines such as NK-92. Moreover, human embryonic stem cell (hESC) and induced pluripotent stem cell (iPSC) were verified to be the new source of functional NK cells.

The hESC and iPS-derived NK cells with a sophisticated approach are relatively new compared with the NK cell from PBMC and or CD34+ cells [73]. Currently, research focused on the optimization of experimental design and culture conditions to generate hESC as well as iPS-derived NK cells [74, 75]. These cells could lyse malignant cells by both direct cell-mediated cytotoxicity and antibody-dependent cytotoxic cell lysis. Kaufmann and co-workers produced mature and functional NK cells from hESC and iPS though IL-21 expressing antigen-presenting cells, it took at least 2 months. And the harvested NK cells were on clinical scale [76].

CARs were developed to equip immune effector cells with the ability to recognize antigens on the surface of tumors and kill their targets in an HLA-unrestricted fashion [77]. CAR is short for chimeric antigen receptor, which is composed of three regions, an extracellular domain, a transmembrane domain, and an intracellular domain. The extracellular domain in CAR-T cells guaranteed the specificity of T cells toward a specific target expressed in tumor cells without antigen presentation. It was derived from the single chain variable fragment (scFV) of a monoclonal antibody (mAb). The intracellular domain would activate the lytic pathway of T cells, which is derived from the T cell receptor (TCR)/CD3 complex. In addition, the co-stimulatory signaling endo-domains (CD28, 4-1BB, or OX40) activate T-cell proliferation after the encounter with the target cell. The number of co-stimulatory domains can differ between the different CARs [78].

CAR-T cell therapy has appeared as a revolutionary immunotherapy option for the treatment of hematological malignancies nowadays, whereas CAR-NK cell is still under development. A large number of activating receptors would initiate NK cell cytotoxic activity, based on this one would hypothesize that NK cells do not need a CAR. However, many negative clinical results regarding NK cells transferred into refractory tumor patients indicated otherwise. NK cell activation can be promoted by augmenting activating signals and down-regulating inhibitory signals through genetic engineering techniques. Nevertheless, the addition of a CAR into NK cells might add another option to recognize tumor cells. Specifically, for patients with down-regulation of the ligands required for activation of NK receptors, CAR was necessary. Furthermore, after recognition of tumor cells, the CAR would induce NK cell expansion and increase NK cell persistence. Recently, a few preclinical studies using CAR-NK cells have been published [79–82]. These studies produced CAR-NK cells targeting CD19 and CD20 for B cell malignancies, targeting CD5 for T cell malignancies, and targeting CD138 and CS1 for multiple myeloma.

As for solid malignancies, many researches have been done to use CAR-NK cells against the tumor. The ErbB2/HER2-specific chimeric antigen receptor was linked to NK cells to target breast cancer and glioblastoma [83, 84]. Disialoganglioside GD2-specific NK cells were engineered to target against drug-resistant neuroblastoma [85]. Genssler et al. have used NK-92 cells, which expressed CARs carrying a composite CD28-CD3ζ domain for signaling, and scFv antibody fragments for cell binding, to recognize EGFR, EGFRvIII, or an epitope common to both antigens, to kill heterogeneous glioblastoma cells [86]. Functional NK cells for adoptive therapy can be derived from several different sources [87]. It was verified that autologous NK cells had limited activity against the patient's own tumor cells since self-HLA molecules inhibited the efficacy of autologous NK cells [88–90]. Liu and co-workers have genetically modified cord blood NK cells with CARs that carry the CD19 gene to redirect specificity to CD19 [91]. These CAR-NK cells ectopically produced IL-15 to promote proliferation and survival. In addition, this CAR carried a suicidal gene, inducible caspase-9 (iC9), in order to eliminate transduced cells whenever needed [92].

The most widely studied NK cell line by far is NK-92 cells, which was originally established from a patient with non-Hodgkin's Lymphoma. The lack of almost all inhibitory KIRs made NK-92 cells have higher anti-tumor activity. NK-92 cells have been engineered to express various CARs such as CD19, CD20, CD38, and CS1 for hematologic malignance, and Her2 for solid tumors [83, 93–95]. CAR-NK-92 cells have also been intratumorally injected, allowing them to traffic to tumor sites and exert their effect *via* a vaccine-like mechanism [96].

The promising results in some studies indicated that the addition of IL15 into the CAR construct would enhance the persistence of NK cells *in vivo* [97]. Moreover, Muller et al. have added the C-X-X motif chemokine receptor 4 (CXCR4) into the CAR to enable NK cells to traffic to tumor sites [98]. Nevertheless, NK-92 cells have inherent drawbacks that must be taken into account, which were the potential tumorigenicity, multiple cytogenetic abnormalities, and latent infection with the Epstein-Barr virus. So it should be irradiated prior to clinical use [99].

Both hESCs and iPSCs-derived NK cells were also suitable for CAR expression, which could be maintained indefinitely to provide an almost limitless supply of NK cells. It was reported that NK cells from cord blood CD34+ cells were modified to express CD19-CAR [100].

2.6 NK cell-based cancer immunotherapy

It was demonstrated that in multiple malignant tumors including acute myeloid leukemia and multiple myeloma, NK cell number, and surface-activating receptors NKp30, NKG2D were downregulated, while the inhibitory receptors were over-expressed [101, 102]. Any activating and inhibitory receptor expression disorders would render NK cells unable to activate normally, the ability to secrete cytokines and chemokines would be inhibited, and the cytotoxicity would be affected. Hence, many efforts have been made to produce "off-the-shelf" NK cells to treat cancers [103–105].

NK cells lead immune surveillance against cancer and early elimination of small tumors. The first clinical use of NK cells involved infusing IL-2-activated lymphokine-activated killer cells (LAK cells)) into cancer patients in the 1980s [106]. And recently, many *in vitro* as well as *in vivo* studies had documented the ability of activated NK cells to kill both hematologic malignancies and solid tumors.

2.6.1 Hematologic malignancy

The therapeutic potential of NK cells has been extensively explored in hematological malignancies. Miller et al. have tested haploidentical, related-donor NK-cell infusions in patients with poor-prognosis acute myeloid leukemia resulting in a marked rise in endogenous IL-15, expansion of donor NK cells, and induction of complete hematologic remission in 5 of 19 poor-prognosis patients with AML [107]. Another study also used haploidentical NK cell transplantation, which was killer immunoglobulin-like receptor-human leukocyte antigen (KIR-HLA)-mismatched NK cells, to treat acute myeloid leukemia in children. It also verified the safety of the NK cells with limited hematologic toxicity and no GVHD. And the 2-year event-free survival estimate was 100% [108]. Liu and co-workers have administered HLA-mismatched anti-CD19 CAR-NK cells derived from cord blood to 11 patients with relapsed or refractory CD19-positive non-Hodgkin's lymphoma or chronic lymphocytic leukemia (CLL). These cells were safe and were not associated with the development of cytokine release syndrome, neurotoxicity, or GVHD. Of the 11 patients who were treated, 8 (73%) had a response, 7 had a complete remission, and 1 had remission of the Richter's transformation component but had persistent CLL. Responses were rapid and seen within 30 days after infusion at all dose levels. The infused CAR-NK cells expanded and persisted at low levels for at least 12 months [109]. Torelli's group has enrolled 103 newly diagnosed acute lymphoblastic leukemia patients with 46 adults and 57 children. Significantly higher expression of Nec-2, ULBP-1, and ULBP-3 was found in the pediatric blasts compared to adult cells. In addition, higher surface expression of NKG2D and DNAM1 ligands was found in BCR-ABL gene fusion group. Accordingly, the BCR-ABL fusion gene group was proved to be significantly more susceptible to NK cell-dependent lysis than the B-lineage group [110]. Moreover, NK cells were used to treat various malignancies, and mixed results were obtained. Shi et al infused haploidentical KIR-mismatched NK cells into 10 patients with relapsed multiple myeloma, followed 14 days later with an autologous stem cell graft. Five patients achieved near complete remission [111]. However, when six non-Hodgkin lymphoma patients were transplanted with infused haploidentical NK cells, the NK cells expanded poorly *in vivo*. Besides, the host regulatory T cells were significantly increased after NK cell infusion and IL-2 administration [112]. Pretreatment with ontak (denileukin diftitox) to deplete host regulatory T cells before NK cell transplantation would get a better result. Bachanova et al. have applied the combined Ontak treatment with infused haploidentical NK cells to AML patients, the NK cell expansion was increased, and the AML clearance was enhanced [113].

2.6.2 Solid malignancy

Tumor cells have developed several mechanisms to overcome the constant immune surveillance, prevent NK cell-induced apoptosis, and diminish the efficacy of NK cell-mediated tumor clearance. And the efficacy of NK cells in solid tumors remains undetermined since the preclinical and clinical data are not enough.

NAGAI and co-workers have enrolled nine patients with metastatic pancreatic, ovarian, colonic, renal, and adenocystic carcinoma to receive intravenously NK cell therapy. The NK cells were obtained from HLA/KIR mismatched healthy donors. The dose was starting from 10^6 to 10^8 cells for each patient at 2-week dosing intervals. The results showed that neither grade 2 or higher toxicities, nor adverse events causing discontinuation of protocol treatment were found after NK cell therapy. When the number of administered NK cells was increased to 10^8 cells in four cases, no serious dose-limiting toxicity was found. The overall response rate was 40%, one with partial response and three with stable disease, and the patient with the partial response is still alive after 4 year's observation [114]. Janneke et al. have summarized the pre-clinical and clinical trials on NK cell immunotherapy in ovarian cancer [115]. In six clinical trials with intravenous infusion of NK cells, only 31 patients have been reported that received NK cell adoptive transfer. The majority of patients reached stable disease after NK cell therapy, with a mild pattern of side effects. More complete responses were found in patients with repeated NK cell infusions.

Some *ex vivo* studies also verified the NK cell efficacy against hepatocellular carcinoma (HCC) cell lines. Kamiya and co-workers have obtained activated NK cells from the peripheral blood of healthy donors with stimulation by K562-mb15-41BBL cell line. The viability of three HCC cell lines was reduced after sorafenib treatment, and after 4 hours of culture with NK cells at 1:1 ET ratio, the viability of HCC cells further decreased twofolds. In addition, they used immune-deficient NOD/SCID IL2RGnull mice engrafted with Hep3B to test the efficacy of NK cells, and it was found that NK cells markedly reduced tumor growth and improved the overall survival of the mice [116]. Bugide et al. have found that HCC cells downregulated NKG2D ligands and were resistant to NK cell-mediated eradication. Thirty-two chemical inhibitors of epigenetic regulators, which were able to re-express NKG2D ligands, were tested to investigate if the HCC cell eradication by NK cells was improved. It was found that the inhibition of EZH2, a transcriptional repressor of NKG2D ligand, by small-molecule inhibitors or genetic means enhanced HCC cell eradication by NK cells in an NKG2D ligand-dependent manner [117].

Xiao et al. have constructed NKG2D RNA CAR-NK cells to enhance the cytolytic activity against several solid tumor cell lines as well as in xenografts. In addition, local infusion of the CAR-NK cells was used to treat three patients with metastatic colorectal cancer. The results showed that the ascites generation of two patients, who were intraperitoneal infusion of low doses of the CAR-NK cells, reduced and tumor cell number in ascites samples was significantly decreased. The other patient with a metastatic tumor site in the liver was treated with intraperitoneal infusion of the CAR-NK cells. Rapid tumor regression in the liver region was observed with Doppler ultrasound imaging and complete metabolic response in the treated liver lesions was confirmed by positron emission tomography (PET)-computed tomographic (CT) scanning [118].

Cancer stem cells (CSCs) are a subpopulation within the tumor, which is capable of self-renewal by asymmetrical cell division [119]. CSCs were considered as the basis of tumor's cellular heterogeneity as well as the main culprit of tumorigenesis, tumor progression, and metastasis. CSCs are resistant to conventional cancer therapies, and their persistence following treatment is strongly believed to drive tumor recurrence [120, 121]. The lack/downregulation of consistent surface markers was found in CSCs including MHC-1 [122]. Nevertheless, CSCs were highly susceptible to NK cell-mediated cytotoxicity [123, 124]. By using multiple preclinical models, including autologous and allogeneic NK coculture with cancer cell lines and dissociated primary cancer specimens, as well as pancreatic cancer xenografts, Ames et al. have demonstrated that activated NK cells were capable of preferentially killing CSCs identified by multiple CSC markers including $CD24^+/CD44^+$, $CD133^+$, and aldehyde dehydrogenase (ALDH) ^{bright} [125]. Similar work involving CSCs has been reported in osteosarcoma [126]. Fernández and co-workers have found osteosarcoma cells were susceptible to NK cells' lysis both *in vivo* and *in vitro*, which relied on the interaction between NKG2D receptor and NKG2D ligands (NKG2DL). Moreover, spironolactone increased the susceptibility of osteosarcoma cells to NK cells and could shrink the osteosarcoma CSCs. Tallerico et al. demonstrated that colorectal CSCs showed increased susceptibility to NK cells, which was associated with the upregulation of the activating natural cytotoxicity receptors Kp30 and NKp44 [127]. Castriconi et al. reported that glioblastoma-derived CSCs were susceptible to NK cell cytotoxicity. Fresh tumor specimens from glioblastoma patients were used. They have found these neural-CSCs were resistant to unactivated NK cells, but were highly susceptible to both allogeneic and autologous NK cells in co-culture models after pre-treatment with IL-2 and IL-15 [128]. It was reported that when melanoma cell lines were exposed to IL-2-activated allogeneic NK cells, both $CD133^-$ non-CSCs and $CD133^+$ CSCs showed sensitivity to NK cell cytotoxicity, which was possibly mediated by the DNAM-1 ligands Nestin-2 and PVR [129]. In breast cancer, CSCs were $CD44^+CD24^-$ subpopulation. It was found that IL-2 and IL-15-activated NK cells could kill breast cancer CSCs mediated by increased expression of the NKG2D ligands such as ULBP1, ULBP2, and MICA on breast CSCs [130].

3. Challenge and future perspective

Allogeneic NK cell treatment against cancer has seen rapid development. Clinical trials of NK cell-based adoptive transfer to treat relapsed or refractory malignancies have used peripheral blood, umbilical cord blood, hESC- and iPSC-derived NK cells, as well as NK cell lines. Although tumors may develop several mechanisms to resist attacks from endogenous NK cells, *ex vivo* activation, expansion, and genetic modification of NK cells can greatly increase their anti-tumor activity and equip them to overcome resistance. Some of these methods have been translated into clinical-grade platforms and support clinical trials of NK cell infusions in patients with hematological malignancies or solid tumors [131, 132]. Surprisingly, many of the clinical studies involving NK cells against tumors did not show optimal results [133]. It was reported that after *in vitro* expansion of NK cells, the KIR-HLA-I mismatch effect in some occasions can be bypassed, and the expression of NK receptors becomes homogenous, which inhibited the killing ability [134].

Effective adoptive NK cell-based immunotherapy requires NK cells to be activated, sufficient in number, and considerably persistent in the body, to enter tumor sites and effectively kill tumor cells. These factors can be co-administered with adoptive cell infusions or the NK cells themselves can be modified to secrete or present membrane-bound factors. IL-15, for example, would increase NK cell persistence *in vivo* [135]. hESC and iPSC-derived NK cells are phenotypically similar to the NK cells in peripheral blood, and they express more KIR compared to umbilical cord blood-derived NK cells, which made them unlimited source for the adoptive transfer of NK cells [73, 136]. On the other hand, the safety of hESC and iPSC-derived NK cells in terms of potential tumorigenicity needs to be determined before they can be utilized in the clinical setup.

Recently, gene-modified NK cells have been successfully developed to possess specific tumor antigens or secreting certain immunosuppressive cytokines to enhance the cytotoxicity of NK cells. Nevertheless, different transduction methods, both viral and non-viral, have been used to modify NK cells, and different expansion strategies were used. So it was difficult to obtain NK cells with homogenous functions. Additionally, lentiviral and retroviral vectors are designed to ensure persistent transgene expression. However, safety remains controversial [137, 138]. Alternatively, non-viral transduction methods, including electroporation, are being explored. Electroporation introduces CAR-encoding mRNA through pores in the cell membrane, resulting in the immediate expression of the CAR molecule. However, mRNA electroporation was reported to result in markedly lower efficiencies [139]. In future studies, more efficient and safe transduction methods should be developed to improve the activity and persistence of NK cells. Moreover, the functional homogenously NK cells should be produced as the "off-the-shell" products.

Conflict of interest

The authors declare no conflict of interest.

Author details

Li Zhang* and Chang Liu
Dalian Municipal Central Hospital Affiliated to Dalian University of Technology, Dalian, China

*Address all correspondence to: tyouri19652004@hotmail.com

References

[1] Smahel M. PD-1/PD-L1 blockade therapy for tumors with downregulated MHC class I expression. International Journal of Molecular Sciences. 2017;**18**:E1331. DOI: 10.3390/ijms18061331

[2] Di Vito C, Mikulak J, Zaghi E, Pesce S, Marcenaro E, Mavilio D. NK cells to cure cancer. Seminars in Immunology. 2019;**41**:101272. DOI: 10.1016/j.smim.2019.03.004

[3] Pesce S, Greppi M, Grossi F, Del Zotto G, Moretta L, Sivori S, et al. PD/1-PD-Ls checkpoint: Insight on the potential role of NK cells. Frontiers in Immunology. 2019;**10**:1242. DOI: 10.3389/fimmu.2019.01242

[4] Minetto P, Guolo F, Pesce S, Greppi M, Obino V, Ferretti E, et al. Harnessing NK cells for cancer treatment. Frontiers in Immunology. 2019;**10**:2836. DOI: 10.3389/fimmu.2019.02836

[5] Herberman RB, Nunn ME, Holden HT, Lavrin DH. Natural cytotoxic reactivity of mouse lymphoid cells against syngeneic and allogeneic tumors. II. Characterization of effector cells. International Journal of Cancer. 1975;**16**:230-239. DOI: 10.1002/ijc.2910160205

[6] Myers JA, Miller JS. Exploring the NK cell platform for cancer immunotherapy. Nature Reviews. Clinical Oncology. 2021;**18**:85-100. DOI: 10.1038/s41571-020-0426-7

[7] Miller JS, Lanier LL. Natural killer cells in cancer immunotherapy. Annual Review in Cancer Biology. 2019;**3**:77-103. DOI: 10.1186/s12943-020-01238-x

[8] Male V, Hughes T, McClory S, Colucci F, Caligiuri MA, Moffett A. Immature NK cells, capable of producing IL-22, are present in human uterine mucosa. Journal of Immunology. 2010;**185**:3913-3918. DOI: 10.4049/jimmunol.1001637

[9] Scoville SD, Freud AG, Caligiuri MA. Modeling human natural killer cell development in the era of innate lymphoid cells. Frontiers in Immunology. 2017;**8**:360. DOI: 10.3389/fimmu.2017.00360

[10] Barton K, Muthusamy N, Fischer C, Ting CN, Walunas TL, Lanier LL, et al. The Ets-1 transcription factor is required for the development of natural killer cells in mice. Immunity. 1998;**9**:555-563. DOI: 10.1016/s1074-7613(00)80638-x

[11] Boggs SS, Trevisan M, Patrene K, Geogopoulos K. Lack of natural killer cell precursors in fetal liver of Ikaros knockout mutant mice. Natural Immunity. 1998;**16**:137-145. DOI: 10.1159/000069438

[12] Morice WG. The immunophenotypic attributes of NK cells and NK-cell lineage lymphoproliferative disorders. American Journal of Clinical Pathology. 2007;**127**:881-886. DOI: 10.1309/Q49CRJ030L22MHLF

[13] Ljunggren HG, Karre K. In search of the 'missing self': MHC molecules and NK cell recognition. Immunology Today. 1990;**11**:237-244. DOI: 10.1016/0167-5699(90)90097-s

[14] Moretta A, Tambussi G, Bottino C, Tripodi G, Merli A, Ciccone E, et al. A novel surface antigen expressed by a subset of human CD3- CD16+ natural killer cells. Role in cell activation and regulation of cytolytic function. The Journal of Experimental Medicine.

1990;**171**:695-714. DOI: 10.1084/jem.171.3.695

[15] Moretta A, Bottino C, Pende D, Tripodi G, Tambussi G, Viale O, et al. Identification of four subsets of human CD3-CD16+ natural killer (NK) cells by the expression of clonally distributed functional surface molecules: Correlation between subset assignment of NK clones and ability to mediate specific alloantigen recognition. The Journal of Experimental Medicine. 1990;**172**:1589-1598. DOI: 10.1084/jem.172.6.1589

[16] Braud VM, Allan DS, O'Callaghan CA, Soderstrom K, D'Andrea A, Ogg GS, et al. HLA-E binds to natural killer cell receptors CD94/NKG2A, B and C. Nature. 1998;**391**:795-799. DOI: 10.1038/35869

[17] Lanier LL. Up on the tightrope: Natural killer cell activation and inhibition. Nature Immunology. 2008;**9**:495-502. DOI: 10.1038/ni1581

[18] Sivori S, Carlomagno S, Pesce S, Moretta A, Vitale M, Marcenaro E. TLR/NCR/KIR: Which one to use and when? Frontiers in Immunology. 2014;**5**:105. DOI: 10.3389/fimmu.2014.00105

[19] Vivier E, Raulet DH, Moretta A, Caligiuri MA, Zitvogel L, Lanier LL, et al. Innate or adaptive immunity? The example of natural killer cells. Science. 2011;**331**:44-49. DOI: 10.1126/science.1198687

[20] Marcenaro E, Dondero A, Moretta A. Multi-directional cross-regulation of NK cell function during innate immune responses. Transplant Immunology. 2006;**17**:16-19. DOI: 10.1016/j.trim.2006.09.019

[21] Martín-Antonio B, Suñe G, Perez-Amill L, Castella M, Urbano-Ispizua A. Natural Killer Cells: Angels and Devils for Immunotherapy. International Journal of Molecular Sciences. 2017;**18**:1868. DOI: 10.3390/ijms18091868

[22] Horowitz A, Strauss-Albee DM, Leipold M, Kubo J, Nemat-Gorgani N, Dogan OC, et al. Genetic and environmental determinants of human NK cell diversity revealed by mass cytometry. Science Translational Medicine. 2013;**5**:208ra145. DOI: 10.1126/scitranslmed.3006702

[23] Di Santo JP. Natural killer cell developmental pathways: A question of balance. Annual Review of Immunology. 2006;**24**:257-286. DOI: 0.1146/annurev.immunol.24.021605.090700

[24] Freud AG, Caligiuri MA. Human natural killer cell development. Immunological Reviews. 2006;**214**:56-72. DOI: 10.1111/j.1600-065X.2006.00451.x

[25] Romagnani C, Juelke K, Falco M, Morandi B, D'Agostino A, Costa R, et al. CD56brightCD16- killer Ig-like receptor-NK cells display longer telomeres and acquire features of CD56dim NK cells upon activation. Journal of Immunology. 2007;**178**:4947-4955. DOI: 10.4049/jimmunol.178.8.4947

[26] Bjorkstrom NK, Riese P, Heuts F, Andersson S, Fauriat C, Ivarsson MA, et al. Malmberg. expression patterns of NKG2A, KIR, and CD57 define a process of CD56dim NK-cell differentiation uncoupled from NK-cell education. Blood. 2010;**116**:3853-3864. DOI: 10.1182/blood-2010-04-281675

[27] Moretta L, Bottino C, Pende D, Vitale M, Mingari MC, Moretta A. Different checkpoints in human NK-cell activation. Trends in Immunology. 2004;**25**:670-676. DOI: 10.1016/j.it.2004.09.008

[28] Andre P, Denis C, Soulas C, Bourbon-Caillet C, Lopez J, Arnoux T, et al. Anti-NKG2A mAb is a checkpoint inhibitor that promotes anti-tumor immunity by unleashing both T and NK cells. Cell. 2018;**175**:1731-1743. DOI: 10.1016/j.cell.2018.10.014

[29] Pesce S, Greppi M, Tabellini G, Rampinelli F, Parolini S, Olive D, et al. Identification of a subset of human natural killer cells expressing high levels of programmed death 1: A phenotypic and functional characterization. The Journal of Allergy and Clinical Immunology. 2017;**139**:335-346. DOI: 10.1016/j.jaci.2016.04.025.

[30] Sun H, Sun C. The rise of NK cell checkpoints as promising therapeutic targets in cancer immunotherapy. Frontiers in Immunology. 2019;**10**:2354. DOI: 10.3389/fimmu.2019.02354

[31] Sivori S, Vacca P, Del Zotto G, Munari E, Mingari MC, Moretta L. Human NK cells: Surface receptors, inhibitory checkpoints, and translational applications. Cellular & Molecular Immunology. 2019;**16**:430-441. DOI: 10.1038/s41423-019-0206-4

[32] Karre K, Ljunggren HG, Piontek G, Kiessling R. Selective rejection of H-2-deficient lymphoma variants suggests alternative immune defence strategy. Nature. 1986;**319**:67-68. DOI: 10.1038/319675a0

[33] Malnati MS, Lusso P, Ciccone E, Moretta A, Moretta L, Long EO. Recognition of virus-infected cells by natural killer cell clones is controlled by polymorphic target cell elements. The Journal of Experimental Medicine. 1993;**178**:961-969. DOI: 10.1084/jem.178.3.961

[34] Bauer S, Groh V, Wu J, Steinle A, Phillips JH, Lanier LL, et al. Activation of NK cells and T cells by NKG2D, a receptor for stress-inducible MICA. Science. 1999;**285**:727-729. DOI: 10.1126/science.285.5428.727

[35] Moretta A. Natural killer cells and dendritic cells: Rendezvous in abused tissues. Nature Reviews. Immunology. 2002;**2**:957-964. DOI: 10.1038/nri956

[36] Lucas M, Schachterle W, Oberle K, Aichele P, Diefenbach A. Dendritic cells prime natural killer cells by trans-presenting interleukin 15. Immunity. 2007;**26**:503-517. DOI: 10.1016/j.immuni.2007.03.006

[37] Li Z, Li D, Tsun A, Li B. FOXP3(+) regulatory T cells and their functional regulation. Cellular & Molecular Immunology. 2015;**12**:558-565. DOI: 10.3389/fimmu.2021.750542

[38] Zhang S, Ke X, Zeng S, Wu M, Lou J, Wu L, et al. Analysis of CD8(+) Treg cells in patients with ovarian cancer: A possible mechanism for immune impairment. Cellular & Molecular Immunology. 2015;**12**:580-591. DOI: 10.1038/cmi.2015.57

[39] Takeda K, Hayakawa Y, Smyth MJ, Kayagaki N, Yamaguchi N, Kakuta S, et al. Involvement of tumor necrosis factor-related apoptosis-inducing ligand in surveillance of tumor metastasis by liver natural killer cells. Nature Medicine. 2001;**7**:94-100. DOI: 10.1038/83416

[40] Vanden Berghe T, Linkermann A, Jouan-Lanhouet S, Walczak H, Vandenabeele P. Regulated necrosis: The expanding network of non-apoptotic cell death pathways. Nature Reviews. Molecular Cell Biology. 2014;**15**:135-147. DOI: 10.1038/nrm3737

[41] Mace EM, Zhang J, Siminovitch KA, Takei F. Elucidation of the integrin LFA-1-mediated signaling pathway of actin polarization in natural killer cells.

Blood. 2010;**116**:1272-1279. DOI: 10.1182/blood-2009-12-261487

[42] Hua G, Wang S, Zhong C, Xue P, Fan Z. Ignition of p53 bomb sensitizes tumor cells to granzyme K-mediated cytolysis. Journal of Immunology. 2009;**182**:215-219. DOI: 10.4049/jimmunol.0802307

[43] Wang H, Sun Q, Wu Y, Wang L, Zhou C, Ma W, et al. Granzyme M expressed by tumor cells promotes chemoresistance and EMT in vitro and metastasis in vivo associated with STAT3 activation. Oncotarget. 2015;**6**:5818-5831. DOI: 10.18632/oncotarget.3461

[44] Lee YH, Martin-Orozco N, Zheng P, Li J, Zhang P, Tan H, et al. Inhibition of the B7-H3 immune checkpoint limits tumor growth by enhancing cytotoxic lymphocyte function. Cell Research. 2017;**27**:1034-1045. DOI: 10.1038/cr.2017.90

[45] Rosenberg SA, Lotze MT, Yang JC, Aebersold PM, Linehan WM, Seipp CA, et al. Experience with the use of high-dose interleukin-2 in the treatment of 652 cancer patients. Annals of Surgery. 1989;**210**:474-484. DOI:10.1097/00000658-198910000-00008

[46] Leong JW, Chase JM, Romee R, Schneider SE, Sullivan RP, Cooper MA, et al. Preactivation with IL-12, IL-15, and IL-18 induces CD25 and a functional high-affinity IL-2 receptor on human cytokine-induced memory-like natural killer cells. Biology of Blood and Marrow Transplantation. 2014;**20**:463-473. DOI: 10.1016/j.bbmt.2014.01.006

[47] Ahn YO, Kim S, Kim TM, Song EY, Park MH, Heo DS. Irradiated and activated autologous PBMCs induce expansion of highly cytotoxic human NK cells in vitro. Journal of Immunotherapy. 2013;**36**:373-381. DOI: 10.1097/CJI.0b013e3182a3430f

[48] Lim O, Lee Y, Chung H, Her JH, Kang SM, Jung MY, et al. GMP compliant, large-scale expanded allogeneic natural killer cells have potent cytolytic activity against cancer cells in vitro and in vivo. PLoS One. 2013;**8**:e53611. DOI: 10.1371/journal.pone.0053611

[49] Fujisaki H, Kakuda H, Shimasaki N, Imai C, Ma J, Lockey T, et al. Expansion of highly cytotoxic human natural killer cells for cancer cell therapy. Cancer Research. 2019;**69**:4010-4017. DOI: 10.1158/0008-5472.CAN-08-3712

[50] Denman CJ, Senyukov VV, Somanchi SS, Phatarpekar PV, Kopp LM, Johnson JL, et al. Membrane-bound IL-21 promotes sustained ex vivo proliferation of human natural killer cells. PLoS One. 2012;7:e30264. DOI: 10.1371/journal.pone.0030264

[51] Gong W, Xiao W, Hu M, Weng X, Qian L, Pan X, et al. Ex vivo expansion of natural killer cells with high cytotoxicity by K562 cells modified to co-express major histocompatibility complex class I chain-related protein A, 4-1BB ligand, and interleukin-15. Tissue Antigens. 2010;**76**:467-475. DOI: 10.1111/j.1399-0039.2010.01535.x

[52] Cooper MA, Fehniger TA, Turner SC, Chen KS, Ghaheri BA, Ghayur T, et al. Human natural killer cells: A unique innate immunoregulatory role for the CD56(bright) subset. Blood. 2001;**97**:3146-3151. DOI: 10.1182/blood.v97.10.3146

[53] Vuletić A, Jovanić I, Jurišić V, Milovanović Z, Nikolić S, Spurnić I, et al. IL-2 And IL-15 induced NKG2D, CD158a and CD158b expression on T, NKT- like and NK cell lymphocyte subsets from regional lymph nodes of melanoma patients. Pathology Oncology

Research. 2020;**26**:223-231. DOI: 10.1007/s12253-018-0444-2

[54] Somanchi SS, Senyukov VV, Denman CJ, Lee DA. Expansion, purification, and functional assessment of human peripheral blood NK cells. Journal of Visualized Experiments. 2011;**48**:2540. DOI: 10.3791/2540

[55] Bishara A, de Santis D, Witt CC, Brautbar C, Christiansen FT, Or R, et al. The beneficial role of inhibitory KIR genes of HLA class I NK epitopes in haploidentically mismatched stem cell allografts may be masked by residual donor-alloreactive T cells causing GVHD. Tissue Antigens. 2004;**63**:204-211. DOI: 10.1111/j.0001-2815.2004.00182.x

[56] Lowe EJ, Turner V, Handgretinger R, Horwitz EM, Benaim E, Hale GA, et al. T-cell alloreactivity dominates natural killer cell alloreactivity in minimally T-cell-depleted HLA-non-identical paediatric bone marrow transplantation. British Journal of Haematology. 2003;**123**:323-326. DOI: 10.1046/j.1365-2141.2003.04604.x

[57] Klingemann H. Challenges of cancer therapy with natural killer cells. Cytotherapy. 2015;**17**:245-249. DOI: 10.1016/j.jcyt.2014.09.007

[58] Brehm C, Huenecke S, Quaiser A, Esser R, Bremm M, Kloess S, et al. IL-2 stimulated but not unstimulated NK cells induce selective disappearance of peripheral blood cells: Concomitant results to a phase I/II study. PLoS One. 2011;**6**:e27351. DOI: 10.1371/journal.pone.0027351

[59] Koehl U, Brehm C, Huenecke S, Zimmermann SY, Kloess S, Bremm M, et al. Clinical grade purification and expansion of NK cell products for an optimized manufacturing protocol. Frontiers in Oncology. 2013;**3**:118. DOI: 10.3389/fonc.2013.00118

[60] Childs RW, Berg M. Bringing natural killer cells to the clinic: Ex vivo manipulation. Hematology. American Society of Hematology. Education Program. 2013;**2013**(1):234-246. DOI: 10.1182/asheducation-2013.1.234

[61] Freud AG, Mundy-Bosse BL, Yu J, Caligiuri MA. The broad spectrum of human natural killer cell diversity. Immunity. 2017;**47**:820-833. DOI: 10.1016/j.immuni.2017.10.008

[62] Kweon S, Phan MT, Chun S, Yu H, Kim J, Kim S, et al. Expansion of Human NK Cells Using K562 Cells Expressing OX40 Ligand and Short Exposure to IL-21. Frontiers in Immunology. 2019;**10**:879. DOI: 10.3389/fimmu.2019.00879

[63] Koehl U, Sörensen J, Esser R, Zimmermann S, Grüttner HP, Tonn T, et al. IL-2 activated NK cell immunotherapy of three children after haploidentical stem cell transplantation. Blood Cells, Molecules & Diseases. 2004;**33**:261-266. DOI: 10.1016/j.bcmd.2004.08.013

[64] de Rham C, Ferrari-Lacraz S, Jendly S, Schneiter G, Dayer JM, Villard J. The proinflammatory cytokines IL-2, IL-15 and IL-21 modulate the repertoire of mature human natural killer cell receptors. Arthritis Research & Therapy. 2007;**9**:R125. DOI: 10.1186/ar2336

[65] Tomala J, Chmelova H, Mrkvan T, Rihova B, Kovar M. In vivo expansion of activated naive CD8+ T cells and NK cells driven by complexes of IL-2 and anti-IL-2 monoclonal antibody as novel approach of cancer immunotherapy. Journal of Immunology. 2009;**183**:4904-4912. DOI: 10.4049/jimmunol.0900284

[66] Wu Z, Xu Y. IL-15R alpha-IgG1-Fc enhances IL-2 and IL-15 antitumor

action through NK and CD8+ T cells proliferation and activation. Journal of Molecular Cell Biology. 2010;**2**:217-222. DOI: 10.1093/jmcb/mjq012

[67] Schönberg K, Fischer JC, Kögler G, Uhrberg M. Neonatal NK-cell repertoires are functionally, but not structurally, biased toward recognition of self HLA class I. Blood. 2011;**117**:5152-5156. DOI: 10.1182/blood-2011-02-334441

[68] Fluevano M, Domogala A, Blundell M, Jackson N, Pedroza-Pacheco I, Derniame S, et al. Frozen cord blood hematopoietic stem cells differentiate into higher numbers of functional natural killer cells in vitro that mobilized hematopoietic stem cells or freshly isolated cord blood hematopoietic stem cells. PLoS One. 2014;**9**:e87086. DOI: 10.1371/journal.pone.0087086

[69] Pinho MJ, Punze M, Sousa M, Barros A. Ex vivo differentiation of natural killer cells from human umbilical cord blood CD34+ progenitor cells. Cell Communication & Adhesion. 2011;**18**:45-55. DOI: 10.3109/15419061.2011.610911

[70] Frias AM, Porada CD, Crapnell KB, Cabral JM, Zanjani ED, Almeida-Porada G. Generation of functional natural killer and dendritic cells in a human stromal- based serum-free culture system designed for cord blood expansion. Experimental Hematology. 2008;**36**:61-68. DOI: 10.1016/j.exphem.2007.08.031

[71] Spanholtz J, Tordoir M, Eissens D, Preijers F, van der Meer A, Joosten I, et al. High log-scale expansion of functional human natural killer cells from umbilical cord blood CD34-positive cells for adoptive cancer immunotherapy. PLoS One. 2011;**5**:e9221. DOI: 10.1371/journal.pone.0009221

[72] Chouaib S, Pittari G, Nanbakhsh A, El Ayoubi H, Amsellem S, Bourhis JH, et al. Improving the outcome of leukemia by natural killer cell-based immunotherapeutic strategies. Frontiers in Immunology. 2014;**5**:95. DOI: 10.3389/fimmu.2014.00095

[73] Woll PS, Grzywacz B, Tian X, Marcus RK, Knorr DA, Verneris MR, et al. Human embryonic stem cells differentiate into a homogeneous population of natural killer cells with potent in vivo antitumor activity. Blood. 2009;**113**:6094-6101. DOI: 10.1182/blood-2008-06-165225

[74] Knorr DA, Bock A, Brentjens RJ, Kaufman DS. Engineered human embryonic stem cell-derived lymphocytes to study in vivo trafficking and immunotherapy. Stem Cells and Development. 2013;**22**:1861-1869. DOI: 10.1089/scd.2012.0608

[75] Becker PS, Suck G, Nowakowska P, Ullrich E, Seifried E, Bader P, et al. Selection and expansion of natural killer cells for NK cell-based immunotherapy. Cancer Immunology, Immunotherapy. 2016;**65**:477-484. DOI: 10.1007/s00262-016-1792-y

[76] Knorr DA, Ni Z, Hermanson D, Hexum MK, Bendzick L, Cooper LJ, et al. Clinical-scale derivation of natural killer cells from human pluripotent stem cells for cancer therapy. Stem Cells Translational Medicine. 2013;**2**:274-283. DOI: 10.5966/sctm.2012-0084

[77] Eshhar Z, Waks T, Gross G, Schindler DG. Specific activation and targeting of cytotoxic lymphocytes through chimeric single chains consisting of antibody-binding domains and the gamma or zeta subunits of the immunoglobulin and T-cell receptors. Proceedings of the National Academy Science USA. 1993;**90**:720-724. DOI: 10.1073/pnas.90.2.720

[78] Dotti G, Savoldo B, Brenner M. Fifteen years of gene therapy based on chimeric antigen receptors: "Are we nearly there yet?". Human Gene Therapy. 2009;**20**:1229-1239. DOI: 10.1089/hum.2009.142

[79] Liu E, Tong Y, Dotti G, Shaim H, Savoldo B, Mukherjee M, et al. Cord blood NK cells engineered to express IL-15 and a CD19-targeted CAR show long-term persistence and potent anti-tumor activity. Leukemia. 2018;**32**:520-531. DOI: 10.1038/leu.2017.226

[80] Shimasaki N, Fujisaki H, Cho D, Masselli M, Lockey T, Eldridge P, et al. clinically adaptable method to enhance the cytotoxicity of natural killer cells against B-cell malignancies. Cytotherapy. 2012;**14**:830-840. DOI: 10.3109/14653249.2012.671519

[81] Chu Y, Hochberg J, Yahr A, Ayello J, van de Ven C, Barth M, et al. Targeting CD20+ Aggressive B-cell Non-Hodgkin Lymphoma by Anti-CD20 CAR mRNA-Modified Expanded Natural Killer Cells In Vitro and in NSG Mice. Cancer Immunology Research. 2015;**3**:333-344. DOI: 10.1158/2326-6066.CIR-14-0114

[82] Jiang H, Zhang W, Shang P, Zhang H, Fu W, Ye F, et al. Transfection of chimeric anti-CD138 gene enhances natural killer cell activation and killing of multiple myeloma cells. Molecular Oncology. 2014;**8**:297-310. DOI: 10.1016/j.molonc.2013.12.001

[83] Schonfeld K, Sahm C, Zhang C, Naundorf S, Brendel C, Odendahl M, et al. Selective inhibition of tumor growth by clonal NK cells expressing an ErbB2/HER2-specific chimeric antigen receptor. Molecular Therapy. 2015;**23**:330-338. DOI: 10.1038/mt.2014.219

[84] Zhang C, Burger MC, Jennewein L, Genssler S, Schonfeld K, Zeiner P, et al. ErbB2/HER2-specific NK cells for targeted therapy of glioblastoma. Journal of the National Cancer Institute. 2016;**108**(5). DOI: 10.1093/jnci/djv375

[85] Seidel D, Shibina A, Siebert N, Wels WS, Reynolds CP, Huebener N, et al. Disialoganglioside-specific human natural killer cells are effective against drug-resistant neuroblastoma. Cancer Immunology, Immunotherapy. 2015;**64**:621-634. DOI: 10.1007/s00262-015-1669-5

[86] Genssler S, Burger MC, Zhang C, Oelsner S, Mildenberger I, Wagner M, et al. Dual targeting of glioblastoma with chimeric antigen receptor-engineered natural killer cells overcomes heterogeneity of target antigen expression and enhances antitumor activity and survival. Oncoimmunology. 2016;**5**:e1119354. DOI: 10.1080/2162402X.2015.1119354

[87] Glienke W, Esser R, Priesner C, Suerth JD, Schambach A, Wels WS, et al. Advantages and applications of CAR-expressing natural killer cells. Frontiers in Pharmacology. 2015;**6**:21. DOI: 10.3389/fphar.2015.00021

[88] Stringaris K, Sekine T, Khoder A, Alsuliman A, Razzaghi B, Sargeant R, et al. Leukemia-induced phenotypic and functional defects in natural killer cells predict failure to achieve remission in acute myeloid leukemia. Haematologica. 2013;**99**:836-847. DOI: 10.3324/haematol.2013.087536

[89] Kloess S, Huenecke S, Piechulek D, Esser R, Koch J, Brehm C, et al. IL-2-activated haploidentical NK cells restore NKG2D-mediated NK-cell cytotoxicity in neuroblastoma patients by scavenging of plasma MICA. European Journal of Immunology. 2010;**40**:3255-3267. DOI: 10.1002/eji.201040568

[90] Raffaghello L, Prigione I, Airoldi I, Camoriano M, Levreri I, Gambini C, et al. Downregulation and/or release of NKG2D ligands as immune evasion strategy of human neuroblastoma. Neoplasia. 2004;**6**:558-568. DOI: 10.1593/neo.04316

[91] Liu E, Tong Y, Dotti G, Savoldo B, Muftuoglu M, Kondo K, et al. Cord blood derived natural killer cells engineered with a chimeric antigen receptor targeting CD19 and expressing IL-15 have long term persistence and exert potent anti-leukemia activity. Blood. 2016;**126**:3091. DOI: 10.1038/leu.2017.226

[92] Di Stasi A, Tey SK, Dotti G, Fujita Y, Kennedy-Nasser A, Martinez C, et al. Inducible apoptosis as a safety switch for adoptive cell therapy. The New England Journal of Medicine. 2011;**365**:1673-1683. DOI: 10.1056/NEJMoa1106152

[93] Romanski A, Uherek C, Bug G, Seifried E, Klingemann H, Wels WS, et al. CD19-CAR engineered NK-92 cells are sufficient to overcome NK cell resistance in B-cell malignancies. Journal of Cellular and Molecular Medicine. 2016;**20**:1287-1294. DOI: 10.1111/jcmm.12810

[94] Boissel L, Betancur M, Wels WS, Tuncer H, Klingemann H. Transfection with mRNA for CD19 specific chimeric antigen receptor restores NK cell mediated killing of CLL cells. Leukemia Research. 2009;**33**:1255-1259. DOI: 10.1016/j.leukres.2008.11.024

[95] Boissel L, Betancur-Boissel M, Lu W, Krause DS, Van Etten RA, Wels WS, et al. Retargeting NK-92 cells by means of CD19- and CD20- specific chimeric antigen receptors compares favorably with antibody-dependent cellular cytotoxicity. OncoImmunology. 2013;**2**:e26527. DOI: 10.4161/onci.26527

[96] Boissel L, Klingemann H, Khan J, Soon-Shiong P. Intra-tumor injection of CAR-engineered NK cells induces tumor regression and protection against tumor re-challenge. Blood. 2016;**128**:466. DOI: 10.1182/blood.V128.22.466.466

[97] Liu E, Tong Y, Dotti G, Shaim H, Savoldo B, Mukherjee M, et al. Cord blood NK cells engineered to express IL-15 and a CD19-targeted CAR show long-term persistence and potent antitumor activity. Leukemia. 2018;**32**:520-531. DOI: 10.1038/leu.2017.226

[98] Muller N, Michen S, Tietze S, Topfer K, Schulte A, Lamszus K, et al. Engineering NK cells modified with an EGFRvIII-specific chimeric antigen receptor to overexpress CXCR4 improves immunotherapy of CXCL12/SDF-1-secreting glioblastoma. Journal of Immunotherapy. 2015;**38**:197-210. DOI: 10.1097/CJI.0000000000000082

[99] Uphoff CC, Denkmann SA, Steube KG, Drexler HG. Detection of EBV, HBV, HCV, HIV-1, HTLV-I and -II, and SMRV in human and other primate cell lines. Journal of Biomedicine & Biotechnology. 2010;**2010**:904767. DOI: 10.1155/2010/904767

[100] Lowe E, Truscott LC, De Oliveira SN. In vitro generation of human NK cells expressing chimeric antigen receptor through differentiation of gene-modified hematopoietic stem cells. Methods in Molecular Biology. 2016;**1441**:241-251. DOI: 10.1007/978-1-4939-3684-7_20

[101] Tang L, Wu J, Li CG, Jiang HW, Xu M, Du M, et al. Characterization of immune dysfunction and identification of prognostic immune-related risk factors in acute myeloid leukemia. Clinical Cancer Research. 2020;**26**:1763-1772. DOI: 10.1158/1078-0432.CCR-19-3003

[102] Konjević G, Vuletić A, Mirjačić Martinović K, Colović N, Čolović M, Jurišić V. Decreased CD161 activating and increased CD158a inhibitory receptor expression on NK cells underlies impaired NK cell cytotoxicity in patients with multiple myeloma. Journal of Clinical Pathology. 216;**2016**:203. DOI: 10.1136/jclinpath-2016-203614

[103] Mahaweni NM, Ehlers FAI, Bos GMJ, Wieten L. Tuning natural killer cell anti-multiple myeloma reactivity by targeting inhibitory signaling via KIR and NKG2A. Frontiers in Immunology. 2018;**9**:2848. DOI: 10.3389/fimmu.2018.02848

[104] Easom NJW, Stegmann KA, Swadling L, Pallett LJ, Burton AR, Odera D, et al. IL-15 overcomes hepatocellular carcinoma-induced NK cell dysfunction. Frontiers in Immunology. 2018;**9**:1009. DOI: 10.3389/fimmu.2018.01009

[105] Tomchuck SL, Leung WH, Dallas MH. Enhanced cytotoxic function of natural killer and CD3+CD56+ cells in cord blood after culture. Biology of Blood and Marrow Transplantation. 2015;**21**:39-49. DOI: 10.1016/j.bbmt.2014.10.014

[106] Rosenberg SA, Lotze MT, Muul LM, Leitman S, Chang AE, Ettinghausen SE, et al. Observations on the systemic administration of autologous lymphokine-activated killer cells and recombinant interleukin-2 to patients with metastatic cancer. The New England Journal of Medicine. 1985;**313**(23):1485-1492. DOI: 10.1056/NEJM198512053132327

[107] Miller JS, Soignier Y, Panoskaltsis-Mortari A, McNearney SA, Yun GH, Fautsch SK, et al. Successful adoptive transfer and in vivo expansion of human haploidentical NK cells in patients with cancer. Blood. 2005;**105**:3051-3057. DOI: 10.1182/blood-2004-07-2974

[108] Rubnitz JE, Inaba H, Ribeiro RC, Pounds S, Rooney B, Bell T, et al. NKAML: A Pilot Study to determine the safety and feasibility of haploidentical natural killer cell transplantation in childhood acute myeloid leukemia. Journal of Clinical Oncology. 2010;**28**:955-959. DOI: 10.1200/JCO.2009.24.4590

[109] Liu E, Marin D, Banerjee P, Macapinlac HA, Thompson P, Basar R, et al. Use of CAR-transduced natural killer cells in CD19-positive lymphoid tumors. The New England Journal of Medicine. 2020;**382**:545-553. DOI: 10.1056/NEJMoa1910607

[110] Torelli GF, Peragine N, Raponi S, Pagliara D, De Propris MS, Vitale A, et al. Recognition of adult and pediatric acute lymphoblastic leukemia blasts by natural killer cells. Haematologica. 2014;**99**:1248-1254. DOI: 10.3324/haematol.2013.101931

[111] Shi J, Tricot G, Szmania S, Rosen N, Garg TK, Malaviarachchi PA, et al. Infusion of haplo-identical killer immunoglobulin-like receptor ligand mismatched NK cells for relapsed myeloma in the setting of autologous stem cell transplantation. British Journal of Haematology. 2008;**143**:641-653. DOI: 10.1111/j.1365-2141.2008.07340.x

[112] Bachanova V, Burns LJ, McKenna DH, Curtsinger J, Panoskaltsis-Mortari A, Lindgren BR, et al. Allogeneic natural killer cells for refractory lymphoma. Cancer Immunology, Immunotherapy. 2010;**59**:1739-1744. DOI: 10.1007/s00262-010-0896-z

[113] Bachanova V, Cooley S, Defor TE, Verneris MR, Zhang B, McKenna DH,

et al. Clearance of acute myeloid leukemia by haploidentical natural killer cells is improved using IL-2 diphtheria toxin fusion protein. Blood. 2014;**123**:3855-3863. DOI: 10.1182/blood-2013-10-532531

[114] Nagai K, Harada Y, Harada H, Yanagihara K, Yonemitsu Y, Miyazaki Y. Highly activated Ex Vivo-expanded natural killer cells in patients with solid tumors in a Phase I/IIa Clinical Study. Anticancer Research. 2020;**40**:5687-5570. DOI: 10.21873/Anticanres.14583

[115] Hoogstad-van Evert JS, Bekkers R, Ottevanger N, Jansen JH, Massuger L, Dolstra H. Harnessing natural killer cells for the treatment of ovarian cancer. Gynecologic Oncology. 2020;**157**:810-816. DOI: 10.1016/j.ygyno.2020.03.020

[116] Kamiya T, Chang YH, Campana D. Expanded and activated natural killer cells for immunotherapy of hepatocellular carcinoma. Cancer Immunology Research. 2016;**4**:574-581. DOI: 10.1158/2326-6066.CIR-15-0229

[117] Bugide S, Green MR, Wajapeyee N. Inhibition of enhancer of zeste homolog 2 (EZH2) induces natural killer cell-mediated eradication of hepatocellular carcinoma cells. Proceedings of the National Academy of Sciences of the United States of America. 2018;**115**:E3509-E3518. DOI: 10.1073/pnas.1802691115

[118] Xiao L, Cen D, Gan H, Sun Y, Huang N, Xiong H, et al. Adoptive transfer of NKG2D CAR mRNA-engineered natural killer cells in colorectal cancer patients. Molecular Therapy. 2019;**27**:1114-1125. DOI: 10.1016/j.ymthe.2019.03.011

[119] Beck B, Blanpain C. Unravelling cancer stem cell potential. Nature Reviews. Cancer. 2013;**13**:727-738. DOI: 10.1038/nrc3597

[120] Sakariassen PO, Immervoll H, Chekenya M. Cancer stem cells as mediators of treatment resistance in brain tumors: Status and controversies. Neoplasia. 2007;**9**:882-892. DOI: 10.1593/neo.07658

[121] Chen J, Li Y, Yu TS, McKay RM, Burns DK, Kernie SG, et al. A restricted cell population propagates glioblastoma growth after chemotherapy. Nature. 2012;**488**(7412):522-526. DOI: 10.1038/nature11287

[122] Nguyen PH, Giraud J, Chambonnier L, Dubus P, Wittkop L, Belleannée G, et al. Characterization of biomarkers of tumorigenic and chemoresistant cancer stem cells in human gastric carcinoma. Clinical Cancer Research. 2017;**23**:1586-1597. DOI: 10.1158/1078-0432.CCR-15-2157

[123] Kozlowska AK, Topchyan P, Kaur K, Tseng HC, Teruel A, Hiraga T, et al. Differentiation by NK cells is a prerequisite for effective targeting of cancer stem cells/poorly differentiated tumors by chemopreventive and chemotherapeutic drugs. Journal of Cancer. 2017;**8**:537-554. DOI: 10.7150/jca.15989

[124] Kaur K, Topchyan P, Kozlowska AK, Ohanian N, Chiang J, Maung PO, et al. Super-charged NK cells inhibit growth and progression of stem-like/poorly differentiated oral tumors in vivo in humanized BLT mice; effect on tumor differentiation and response to chemotherapeutic drugs. OncoImmunology. 2018;**7**:e1426518. DOI: 10.1080/2162402X.2018.1426518

[125] Ames E, Canter RJ, Grossenbacher SK, Mac S, Chen M, Smith RC, et al. NK cells preferentially target tumor cells with a cancer stem cell phenotype. Journal of Immunology.

2015;**195**:4010-4019. DOI: 10.4049/jimmunol.1500447

[126] Fernandez L, Valentın J, Zalacain M, Leung W, Patino-Garcıa A, Perez-Martınez A. Activated and expanded natural killer cells target osteosarcoma tumor initiating cells in an NKG2D-NKG2DL dependent manner. Cancer Letters. 2015;**368**:54-63. DOI: 10.1016/j.canlet.2015.07.042

[127] Tallerico R, Todaro M, Di Franco S, Maccalli C, Garofalo C, Sottile R, et al. Human NK cells selective targeting of colon cancer-initiating cells: A role for natural cytotoxicity receptors and MHC class I molecules. Journal of Immunology. 2013;**190**:2381-2390. DOI: 10.4049/jimmunol.1201542

[128] Castriconi R, Daga A, Dondero A, Zona G, Poliani PL, Melotti A, et al. NK cells recognize and kill human glioblastoma cells with stem cell-like properties. Journal of Immunology. 2009;**182**:3530-3539. DOI: 10.4049/jimmunol.0802845

[129] Pietra G, Manzini C, Vitale M, Balsamo M, Ognio E, Boitano M, et al. Natural killer cells kill human melanoma cells with characteristics of cancer stem cells. International Immunology. 2009;**21**:793-801. DOI: 10.1093/intimm/dxp047

[130] Yin T, Wang G, He S, Liu Q, Sun J, Wang Y, et al. Human cancer cells with stem cell-like phenotype exhibit enhanced sensitivity to the cytotoxicity of IL-2 and IL-15 activated natural killer cells. Cellular Immunology. 2016;**300**:41-45. DOI: 10.1016/j.cellimm.2015.11.009

[131] Ciurea SO, Kongtim P, Soebbing D, Trikha P, Behbehani G, Rondon G, et al. Decrease post-transplant relapse using donor-derived expanded NK-cells. Leukemia. 2022;**36**:155-164. DOI: 10.1038/s41375-021-01349-4

[132] Lee SC, Shimasaki N, Lim JSJ, Wong A, Yadav K, Yong WP, et al. Phase I Trial of Expanded, Activated Autologous NK-cell Infusions with Trastuzumab in Patients with HER2-positive Cancers. Clinical Cancer Research. 2020;**26**:4494-4502

[133] Rennert C, Tauber C, Fehrenbach P, Heim K, Bettinger D, Sogukpinar Ö, et al. Adaptive subsets limit the anti-tumoral NK-cell activity in hepatocellular carcinoma. Cell. 2021;**10**:1369. DOI: 10.3390/cells10061369

[134] Huenecke S, Zimmermann SY, Kloess S, Esser R, Brinkmann A, Tramsen L, et al. IL-2-driven regulation of NK cell receptors with regard to the distribution of CD16+ and CD16- subpopulations and in vivo influence after haploidentical NK cell infusion. Journal of Immunotherapy. 2010;**33**:200-210. DOI: 10.1097/CJI.0b013e3181bb46f7

[135] Zhang M, Wen B, Anton OM, Yao Z, Dubois S, Ju W, et al. IL-15 enhanced antibody-dependent cellular cytotoxicity mediated by NK cells and macrophages. Proceedings of the National Academy of Sciences of the United States of America. 2018;**115**:E10915-E10924. DOI: 10.1073/pnas.1811615115

[136] Siegler EL, Zhu Y, Wang P, Yang L. Off-the-shelf CAR-NK cells for cancer immunotherapy. Cell Stem Cell. 2018;**23**:160-161. DOI: 10.1016/j.stem.2018.07.007

[137] Cockrell AS, Kafri T. Gene delivery by lentivirus vectors. Molecular Biotechnology. 2007;**36**:184-204. DOI: 10.1007/s12033-007-0010-8

[138] Everson EM, Trobridge GD. Retroviral vector interactions with hematopoietic cells. Current Opinion in Virology. 2016;**21**:41-46. DOI: 10.1016/j.coviro.2016.07.010

[139] Takei Y, Nemoto T, Mu P, Fujishima T, Ishimoto T, Hayakawa Y, et al. In vivo silencing of a molecular target by short interfering RNA electroporation: Tumor vascularization correlates to delivery efficiency. Molecular Cancer Therapeutics. 2008;**7**:211-221. DOI: 10.1158/1535-7163

Chapter 3

Advances in Natural Killer Cells and Immunotherapy for Gastric Cancer

Shixun Ma, Li Li, Jintang Yin, Xiaohu Wang, Chongya Yang, Leisheng Zhang, Tiankang Guo and Hui Cai

Abstract

Gastric cancer is one of the common malignant tumors in the gastrointestinal tract, and the treatment of gastric cancer includes the main ways such as radical resection, adjuvant chemotherapy, palliative care, and drug therapy; however, patients often have defects such as high recurrence rate, high treatment burden, and serious side effects, which impose a heavy burden on the economic and social construction and patients' families. In recent years, novel gastric cancer treatment methods featuring tumor immunotherapy have provided new treatment strategies to improve the above-mentioned defects and increase the cure rate of patients. Natural killer cells (NK cells) are key components of the body's intrinsic immune response and can participate in both the intrinsic and adaptive immune responses, exercising the functions of tumor killing, removing pathogenic microorganisms or abnormal cells and enhancing immunity, and thus have broad prospects for new drug development and clinical treatment. This article reviews the biological properties and functions of NK cells and their interrelationship with gastric cancer treatment, and provides a reference for clinical research.

Keywords: NK cells, gastric cancer, immunotherapy, progress

1. Introduction

Globally, the mortality rate of gastric cancer is high, with approximately 14.3/100,000 in men and 6.9/100,000 in women, with men being higher than women [1, 2]. There are significant geographical differences in the incidence of gastric cancer: it is highest in East Asia, Eastern Europe and South America and lowest in northern and southern Africa. Advanced gastric cancer can metastasise to the liver, pancreas, intestinal ducts, peritoneum, mesentery, greater omentum, esophagus, bile ducts, pelvis and lymph nodes, making treatment outcomes poor. Early diagnosis and early intervention are therefore crucial. The usual treatment for gastric cancer includes the main routes of surgery, chemotherapy and radiotherapy.

However, it often has drawbacks such as high recurrence rate, heavy treatment burden and side effects, which impose a heavy burden on society, economy and patients' families. In recent years, novel gastric cancer treatments featuring tumor immunotherapy have provided new treatment strategies to improve the above-mentioned defects and increase the cure rate of patients [3, 4]. The natural killer cell (NK) is a key cell in the body's innate immune response. It is composed of a unique group of innate lymphocytes that can participate in both the innate and adaptive immune responses and has the intrinsic ability to recognize and eliminate virally infected and tumor cells [5–9]. NK cells play a key role in anti-cancer immunity due to their cytotoxic mechanisms and immune response modulating ability. 20 years ago, NK cells showed good safety and efficacy in the treatment of patients with advanced leukemia [10–13]. Studies suggest that NK cell content and phenotype are significantly altered in patients with a variety of malignant hematological tumors (AML, MDS) and metastatic solid tumors (gastric cancer, lung cancer). This evidence suggests that NK cells have important research value in the management of a wide range of tumors. In recent years, with the paradigm shift and technological advances in chimeric antigen receptor (CAR) engineered passaged T cell therapy, there is confidence in NK cells as a new tool for immunotherapy. Strategies to develop NK cell-based therapies focus on enhancing the potency and persistence of NK cells through co-stimulation of signaling, checkpoint inhibition, and cytokine armor, and aim to specifically redirect NK cells to tumors through CAR expression or using splice molecules. Notably, clinical studies have shown that the proportion of NK cells in the peripheral blood of patients with stage III and IV gastric cancer is significantly lower ($P < 0.05$). In the clinical setting, the promising results of the first generation of NK cell therapies, which showed encouraging efficacy and a remarkable safety profile, have inspired great enthusiasm for continued innovation [14–19]. In this paper, we review the biological properties and functions of NK cells in gastric cancer patients and their interrelationship with gastric cancer therapy, as well as the latest research progress in gastric cancer immunotherapy, to provide a reference for clinical research.

2. Tumor biological characteristics of gastric cancer

2.1 Epidemiological characteristics of gastric cancer

Gastric cancer is one of the most common tumors of the digestive tract and one of the more common cancers in terms of cancer-related morbidity and mortality worldwide. According to the latest statistics gastric cancer is the fourth most common cancer worldwide and the second most common cause of cancer death [20–22]. The treatment of gastric cancer is still based on a combination of surgical procedures. For patients with early-stage gastric cancer, the 5-year overall survival (OS) rate after treatment is 90%. However, approximately 50% of patients are already progressive at diagnosis, with approximately 40–60% of those who undergo radical resection experiencing recurrence. Approximately 30–35% of patients with gastric cancer present with distant metastases at diagnosis, yet R0 resection is unlikely to be achieved in those with peritoneal dissemination. Even when resection of metastases is feasible, patients with metastatic gastric cancer have an extremely high recurrence rate. For such patients, palliative systemic therapy is the gold standard, and median survival rarely exceeds 12 months [23–30].

2.2 Risk factors for gastric cancer

Risk factors for gastric cancer include a number of aspects including geographical environment, dietary lifestyle, *Helicobacter pylori* (Hp) infection, precancerous lesions and genetics [31–34]. There are significant geographical differences in the development of gastric cancer. Smoking, nitrites, fungal toxins and polycyclic aromatic hydrocarbon compounds are the main carcinogens in terms of dietary life. *H. pylori* infection is a biological causative factor in the development of gastric cancer. Gastric polyps, chronic atrophic gastritis and residual stomach after partial gastrectomy are lesions that may be associated with varying degrees of chronic inflammatory processes, intestinal epithelial metaplasia or atypical hyperplasia of the gastric mucosa, with the potential for transformation into cancer. Genetic and molecular biology studies have shown that the incidence of gastric cancer is four times higher in blood relatives of gastric cancer patients than in controls. The carcinogenesis of gastric cancer is a multifactorial, multi-step and multi-stage development process involving changes in oncogenes, oncogenes, apoptosis-related genes and metastasis-related genes, and the forms of genetic changes are also varied [35–37].

2.3 Tumor microenvironment

The tumor microenvironment (TME) is the internal and external environment in which tumourigenesis, growth and metastasis are associated with tumor cells. It contains cancer cells, stromal cells and macrophages, a large number of immune cells and cells secreting factors that are recruited from a distance. Through their autocrine and paracrine actions, they alter and maintain the conditions for their own survival and development, and promote tumor growth and development. Systemic and local tissues can also limit and influence tumor development and progression through metabolic, secretory, immune, structural and functional alterations [38–41]. In recent years, the tumor immune microenvironment has played a key role in the development of gastric cancer. The immune system recognizes cancer cells and inhibits tumor development and metastasis.. However, tumor cells evade immune attack and induce immunosuppressive TME through two main pathways. Firstly, cancer cells hide the expression of surface antigens to avoid recognition by cytotoxic T cells. Secondly, immune tolerance to TME is induced by the secretion of immunosuppressive molecules such as interleukin-10 and VEGF [42–44].

2.4 Importance of the immune system in gastric cancer

The development, progression and prognosis of gastric cancer are strongly related to the function of the immune system. The common immune cell components in gastric cancer tissues include T cells, B cells, DC cells, NK cells, macrophages M1 and M2, etc. [45–47]. T lymphocytes are derived from lymphatic stem cells from bone marrow, which are differentiated and matured in the thymus, and then distributed to immune organs and tissues throughout the body through lymphatic and blood circulation to perform cellular immune functions. B cells can differentiate into plasma cells when stimulated by antigens, which synthesize and secrete antibodies (immunoglobulins) and perform humoral immunity. Dendritic cells are the body's most powerful and specialized antigen presenting cells (APC), which are highly efficient in the uptake, processing and presentation of antigens. Natural killer cells are derived from bone marrow lymphoid stem cells, which depend on the bone marrow and thymic microenvironment for their differentiation and development, and are mainly found in the bone marrow, peripheral blood, liver, spleen, lung and lymph nodes; NK cells, unlike T and B cells, lymphocytes of tumor cells and virus-infected cells, are a class of non-specific killer cells that do not require pre-sensitisation. Macrophages are differentiated from monocytes in the blood after they have penetrated blood vessels. Infection and chronic inflammation are key factors in the pathogenesis of gastric cancer, with *H. pylori* and other pathogens disrupting the M1 macrophage response, thereby inducing an M2-like activation state, which increases the risk of disease progression [48–52].

3. Relationship between NK cells and gastric cancer

3.1 Biological properties of NK cells

Natural killer cells are important immune cells in the body, not only in the fight against tumors, viral infections and immune regulation, but also in the development of hypersensitivity reactions and autoimmune diseases in some cases, being able to recognize target cells and kill mediators [53]. In the innate immune system, NK cells are specialized immune effector cells that are the first line of anti-tumor lymphocytes and play an important role in tumor immunosurveillance. In previous clinical studies, it has been shown that low NK cell activity correlates with higher tumor incidence and high metastasis rates. nK cells are cytotoxic to tumor cells without prior activation and can modulate various immune responses by secreting immunomodulatory cytokines and chemokines. The combination of activating and inhibiting signals regulates the antitumor effects of NK cells [54]. NK cells are mainly differentiated from CD34+ bone marrow progenitor cells and are mostly present in peripheral blood accounting for 5–10% of PBMC, while active NK are also present in lymph nodes and bone marrow but at lower levels than in peripheral blood [55]. NK cells function differently from T cells and NKT cells due to the lack of expression of TCR and CD3-related complexes. Based on the expression of surface proteins CD56 and CD16, NK cells can be divided into two categories: CD56 + CD16- (immunomodulatory, cytokine production) and CD56-CD16+ (cytotoxic). However, recent advances in high-throughput sequencing and single-cell proteogenomics have revealed that NK cells may exhibit greater phenotypic heterogeneity outside of these two subpopulations, leading to the differentiation of distinct cell populations with different cellular functions [56].

3.2 Functions of NK cells

3.2.1 Cytotoxic functions of NK cells

The killing activity of NK cells is called natural killing activity because it is not restricted by MHC and does not depend on antibodies. NK cells are rich in cytoplasm and contain large asplenophilic granules, the amount of which is positively correlated with the killing activity of NK cells, which appear early after the action of NK cells on target cells, with killing effects seen in vitro at 1 hour and in vivo at 4 hours [57]. NK cells are highly cytotoxic and trigger an effective response by releasing cytolytic particles and cytotoxic cytokines after forming an immune synapse with a target.

The main mediators of killing are perforin, NK cytotoxic factor and TNF. In addition, they can recognize antibody-coated cellular γRIIIA (CD16) receptors via Fc and trigger antibody-dependent cytotoxicity (ADCC) and cytokine production. Killer cell immunoglobulin-like receptors (KIR) and natural killer group 2A (NKG2A) are two major inhibitory receptors that recognize HLA molecules [58, 59].

3.2.2 Immunomodulatory functions of NK cells

NK cells can synthesize and secrete a variety of cytokines to directly kill target cells and are also able to influence the function of B cells, T cells, dendritic cells, macrophages and neutrophils through the production of chemokines. These properties pave the way for it to play a key role in immunotherapy [60].

3.2.3 Memory function of NK cells

Natural killer cells play an important anti-tumor and anti-viral role in vivo, and recent studies have revealed that NK cells have acquired immune cell characteristics and are capable of forming immune memories. NK cell development, differentiation, homeostatic maintenance and memory formation are therefore essential for the implementation of NK cell function [61]. Early studies reported a similar memory response of NK cells in mouse models of cytomegalovirus infection, a behavior not normally associated with innate immune cells. In these studies, when stimulated with a combination of IL-12 and IL-18, mouse NK cells acquired a functional phenotype characterized by increased IFN production γ. Interestingly, after a resting phase, these cells were able to reactivate with the involvement of cytokine stimulation or activation receptors and exhibited enhanced IFNγ-like responses resembling the memory-like properties of adaptive immune cells. Later, Todd Fehniger's group hypothesized that human NK cells should similarly have memory-like properties. Consistent with this hypothesis, their studies showed that human NK cells pre-activated with IL-12, IL-15 and IL-18 and then rested for 1–3 weeks were able to generate a strong response driven by enhanced IFNγ produced after subsequent exposure to cytokines or K562 leukemia cells. Since then, additional research groups have described similar memory-like functions in various immune settings, including the observation of such responses in humans [62, 63].

3.3 Rationale of NK cell anti-tumor

NK cells may have a more important role in immune surveillance and killing of mutated tumor cells than T cells. Patients with certain diseases, such as Chediak-Higashi or X-linked lymphoproliferative syndrome, are particularly susceptible to malignant lymphoproliferative diseases due to a deficiency in NK function [64]. The essence of tumor immunotherapy is to enhance the surveillance and clearance of tumor cells by the patient's immune system through various means [65]. T cells and natural killer (NK) cells are the two most important effector cells that recognize and destroy tumor cells. Precise recognition of both positive signals provided by tumor antigens and negative signals provided by immune checkpoints can be used to determine tumor-specific T-cell activation. Similarly, NK cell activation is dependent on the integration of activating and inhibiting signals. Thus, disrupting the balance by blocking negative and enhancing positive signals from T and NK cells may be beneficial for cancer patients [66]. To date, many therapies have been reported for blocking T and NK cell inhibitory receptors, such as the checkpoint molecules CTLA-4 or PD-1/PD-L1. However, some evidence suggests that these strategies provide benefit to only a limited number of patients with tumors and that most patients continue to experience disease progression. To date, strategies to enhance the anti-tumor function of T cells and NK cells have yielded encouraging results. As the understanding of neoantigens presented by MHC molecules expands, research and clinical implementation of neoantigen-based therapies, including peripatetic T-cell therapies and cancer vaccines, are full of potential for clinical application [67]. The synergistic action of many NK cell surface receptors determines the NK cell state. Tumor cells can be made "invisible" to NK cells by up-regulating inhibitory signals or/and down-regulating activation signals on NK cells, and NK cell function can even be altered by altering the affinity of KIR-MHC interactions through different peptide libraries provided by MHC molecules. Interfering with activating and inhibiting signals has been used in a variety of therapeutic techniques to enhance NK cell function. However, changes in the affinity of the KIR-peptide/MHC complex interactions may occur due to different components of the peptides provided by MHC molecules in tumor cells and may require more research [68].

3.4 Application of NK cells in the treatment of gastric cancer

In gastric cancer patients, NK cells usually exhibit a dysfunctional phenotype characterized by an altered gene expression profile and reduced cytotoxic function, which reduces the feasibility of autologous NK cell therapeutic applications. In addition, the reduced number of autologous NK cells is a major cause of tumor progression. Current NK cell therapy relies on allogeneic sources, namely peripheral blood mononuclear cells, umbilical cord blood, immortalized cell lines, hematopoietic stem and progenitor cells (HSPC) and induced pluripotent stem cells (iPSC). All sources can provide clinically meaningful doses of cells suitable for CAR recipient engineering and have transitioned to human studies. However, they have unique advantages and challenges, and may have different potential transcriptional, phenotypic, and functional properties [69].

3.4.1 NK-92 cells

NK-92, the first NK cell-based immunotherapy to receive U.S. Food and Drug Administration (FDA) clinical trial approval, is a homogenous immortalized NK lymphoma cell line that can be expanded ex vivo to achieve large cell numbers. It was found that NK-92 cells can kill tumor cell lines and primary tumor cells cultured in vitro, and in addition they are not susceptible to immunosuppression, making them promising for tumor cell therapy. However, its oncogenic risk and lack of ADCC-mediated cell killing ability have limited its application [70].

3.4.2 NK cells after in vitro differentiation of CD34+ progenitor cells

Dolstra et al. showed in their trial that transfer of HSPC-NK cells into elderly patients with acute myelogenous leukemia (AML) resulted in better outcomes. However, the safety and efficacy of its application in other tumors needs further validation. Future work will also need to address whether HSPC-NK cells can be effectively designed to achieve enhanced tumor specificity [71].

3.4.3 NK cells after differentiation of iPSCs

Induced pluripotent stem cells (iPSCs) have played an important role in disease modeling, drug discovery and cell therapy, and have contributed to the development of the disciplines of cell biology and regenerative medicine. Currently, iPSCs technology has become an important tool in the study of pathological mechanisms, new drugs are being developed using iPSCs technology, and the number of clinical trials using iPSCs-derived cells is growing. iPSCs are an attractive source of NK cells because of their clonal growth and high expansion capacity, as well as their ability to differentiate in vitro, allowing the manufacture of a large number of homogeneous NK cell products. A potential drawback is that iPSC-derived NK cells typically express low levels of endogenous CD16, although this can be mitigated by genetic engineering. Another possible concern is that iPSCs may have a DNA methylation profile consistent with their somatic cellular tissue origin. This "epigenetic memory" may affect the development of specific cell lineages that differ from the donor cells and should be considered when using iPSC platforms. Nevertheless, a growing number of genetically engineered iPSC-NK cell candidates are emerging from preclinical studies, some of which have already transitioned to clinical trials [72].

3.4.4 NK cells from peripheral blood or from umbilical cord blood

Primary NK cells can be collected from peripheral blood (PB-NK cells) or from umbilical cord blood (CB-NK cells.) CB-NK cells can be readily available frozen through blood banks, whereas PB-NK cells require single harvest and donor-specific collection from healthy donors. in 2005, in work led by Dario Campana, PB-NK cells served as the first successful CAR construct platform for somatic introduction into NK cells, and today, PB-NK cells provide the basis for a variety of current products [73].

4. Conclusion

Immunotherapy is a novel and effective therapeutic strategy that has emerged as a new hope for many patients with gastric cancer. Although NK cell-based immunotherapy is considered to be a safe off-the-shelf antitumor therapy, important issues remain resolved and still a large proportion of gastric cancer patients do not benefit from immunotherapeutic agents. With the development of immunotherapy, it will be important to study the abnormal alterations in the biological phenotype and transcriptomic profile of NK cells, the NK cell subsets and their interrelationship with the prognosis of gastric cancer patients, and to elucidate the key parameters that determine the potency and persistence of NK cells. In addition, to maximize the lifespan and expand the efficacy of NK cells, multiple therapeutic strategies need to be combined [74]. Finally, to ensure NK cell quality, methods for NK cell proliferation and preservation need to be optimized. We believe that great breakthroughs will be achieved in the future in the study of NK cells for immunotherapy of gastric cancer.

Acknowledgements

The authors would like to thank the members in National Postdoctoral Research Station of Gansu Provincial Hospital, Institute of Biology & Hefei Institute of

Physical Science, Chinese Academy of Sciences, and Institute of Health-Biotech, Health-Biotech (Tianjin) Stem Cell Research Institute Co., Ltd. for their technical support. We also thank the staff in Beijing Yunwei Biotechnology Development Co., LTD for their language editing service. This study was supported by the following fund projects: Key Laboratory of Gastrointestinal Tumor Diagnosis and Treatment of National Health and Health Commission (2019PT320005); the National Natural Science Foundation of China (82260031); Key Laboratory of Molecular Diagnosis and Precision Therapy of Surgical Tumors in Gansu Province (18JR2RA033); Gansu Provincial Key Talent Project of Gansu Provincial Party Committee Organization Department (2020RCXM076); Basic Research Innovation Group of Gansu Province (22JR5RA709); Natural Science Foundation of Gansu Province (21JR11RA186, 20JR10RA415); Gansu Provincial Hospital Intra-Hospital Research Fund Project (21GSSYB-8, 20GSSY5-2); The 2021 Central-Guided Local Science and Technology Development Fund (ZYYDDFFZZJ-1); China Postdoctoral Science Foundation (2019 M661033), Science and technology projects of Guizhou Province (QKH-J-ZK[2021]-107), the National Science and Technology Major Projects of China for "Major New Drugs Innovation and Development" (2014ZX09508002-003), Major Program of the National Natural Science Foundation of China (81330015), the project Youth Fund funded by Shandong Provincial Natural Science Foundation (ZR2020QC097), Natural Science Foundation of Tianjin (19JCQNJC12500), Jiangxi Provincial Novel Research & Development Institutions of Shangrao City (2020AB002), Jiangxi Provincial Natural Science Foundation (20224BAB206077, 20212BAB216073), Jiangxi Provincial Key New Product Incubation Program from Technical Innovation Guidance Program of Shangrao City (2020G002).

Conflict of interest

The authors declare no conflict of interest.

Notes/thanks/other declarations

Not applicable.

Appendices and nomenclature

NK cells	natural killer cells
AML	acute myeloid leukemia
MDS	myelodysplastic syndromes
CAR	chimeric antigen receptor
OS	overall survival
EBV	Epstein-Barr virus
MSI	microsatellite instability
MMR	mismatch repair
TME	tumor microenvironment
Tregs	regulatory T cells
MDSCs	myeloid-derived suppressor cells
CTLA-4	cytotoxic T lymphocyte-associated protein 4

PD-1	programmed death protein 1
PD-L1	programmed cell death ligand-1
TIM-3	T cell immunoglobulin and mucin-containing structural domain 3
ADCC	antibody-dependent cytotoxicity
KIR	Killer cell immunoglobulin-like receptors
NKG2A	natural killer group 2A
ITIM	immunoreceptor tyrosine-based inhibitory motifs
HSPC	hematopoietic stem and progenitor cells
FDA	Food and Drug Administration
PB-NK cells	peripheral blood NK cells
CB-NK cells	umbilical cord blood NK cells

Author details

Shixun Ma[1†], Li Li[1†], Jintang Yin[2], Xiaohu Wang[1], Chongya Yang[3], Leisheng Zhang[1,4,5,6*], Tiankang Guo[1*] and Hui Cai[1*]

1 Key Laboratory of Molecular Diagnostics and Precision Medicine for Surgical Oncology in Gansu Province and NHC Key Laboratory of Diagnosis and Therapy of Gastrointestinal Tumor, Gansu Provincial Hospital, Lanzhou, China

2 Department of Clinical Laboratory, Jiuquan Central Blood Station, Jiuquan, China

3 Department of Geriatrics, Lintao County Hospital of Traditional Chinese Medicine, Dingxi, China

4 Jiangxi Research Center of Stem Cell Engineering, Jiangxi Health-Biotech Stem Cell Technology Co., Ltd., Shangrao, China

5 CAS Key Laboratory of Radiation Technology and Biophysics in Institute of Biology & Hefei Institute of Physical Science, Chinese Academy of Sciences, Hefei, China

6 Institute of Health-Biotech, Health-Biotech (Tianjin) Stem Cell Research Institute Co., Ltd, Tianjin, China

*Address all correspondence to: leisheng_zhang@163.com; tiankangguo2020@163.com and caialonteam@163.com

† Co-first author.

References

[1] Waldum HL, Fossmark R: Types of gastric carcinomas. International Journal of Molecular Sciences. 2018;**19**(12):4109

[2] Yeoh KG, Tan P. Mapping the genomic diaspora of gastric cancer. Nature Reviews. Cancer. 2022;**22**(2):71-84

[3] Wrona E, Borowiec M, Potemski P. CAR-NK cells in the treatment of solid tumors. International Journal of Molecular Sciences. 2021;**22**(11):5899

[4] Zhang L, Meng Y, Feng X, Han Z. CAR-NK cells for cancer immunotherapy: From bench to bedside. Biomarker Research. 2022;**10**(1):12

[5] Galon J, Angell HK, Bedognetti D, Marincola FM. The continuum of cancer immunosurveillance: Prognostic, predictive, and mechanistic signatures. Immunity. 2013;**39**(1):11-26

[6] Kennedy LB, Salama AKS. A review of cancer immunotherapy toxicity. CA: a Cancer Journal for Clinicians. 2020;**70**(2):86-104

[7] Vivier E. What is natural in natural killer cells? Immunology Letters. 2006;**107**(1):1-7

[8] Zhang L, Liu M, Yang S, Wang J, Feng X, Han Z. Natural killer cells: Of-the-shelf cytotherapy for cancer immunosurveillance. American Journal of Cancer Research. 2021;**11**(4):1770-1791

[9] Xia J, Minamino S, Kuwabara K. CAR-expressing NK cells for cancer therapy: A new hope. Bioscience Trends. 2020;**14**(5):354-359

[10] Stewart OA, Wu F, Chen Y. The role of gastric microbiota in gastric cancer. Gut Microbes. 2020;**11**:1220-1230

[11] Liu H, Shin SH, Chen H, et al. CDK12 and PAK2 as novel therapeutic targets for human gastric cancer. Theranostics. 2020;**10**:6201-6215

[12] Zhang Y, Zhao J, Yu H, et al. Detection and isolation of free cancer cells from ascites and peritoneal lavages using optically induced electrokinetics (OEK). Science Advances. 2020;**6**:eaba9628

[13] Jie M, Wu Y, Gao M, et al. CircMRPS35 suppresses gastric cancer progression via recruiting KAT7 to govern histone modification. Molecular Cancer. 2020;**19**:56

[14] Tao X, Cheng L, Li Y, et al. Expression of CRYAB with the angiogenesis and poor prognosis for human gastric cancer. Medicine. 2019;**98**:e17799

[15] Ikenoyama Y, Hirasawa T, Ishioka M, et al. Detecting early gastric cancer: Comparison between the diagnostic ability of convolutional neural networks and endoscopists. Digestive Endoscopy. 2021;**33**:141-150

[16] Biagioni A, Skalamera I, Peri S, et al. Update on gastric cancer treatments and gene therapies. Cancer Metastasis Reviews. 2019;**38**:537-548

[17] Toyoshima O, Nishizawa T, Koike K. Endoscopic Kyoto classification of helicobacter pylori infection and gastric cancer risk diagnosis. World Journal of Gastroenterology. 2020;**26**:466-477

[18] Joshi SS, Badgwell BD. Current treatment and recent progress in gastric cancer. CA: a Cancer Journal for Clinicians. 2021;**71**:264-279

[19] Choi IJ, Kim CG, Lee JY, et al. Family history of gastric cancer and helicobacter pylori treatment. New England Journal of Medicine. 2020;**382**:427-436

[20] Chi Y, Wang H, Wang F, et al. PHTF2 regulates lipids metabolism in gastric cancer. Aging. 2020;**12**:6600-6610

[21] Petryszyn P, Chapelle N, Matysiak-Budnik T. Gastric cancer: Where are we heading? Digestive Diseases. 2020;**38**:280-285

[22] Machlowska J, Maciejewski R, Sitarz R. The pattern of signatures in gastric cancer prognosis. International Journal of Molecular Sciences. 2018;**19**:1658

[23] Sundar R, Huang KK, Qamra A, et al. Epigenomic promoter alterations predict for benefit from immune checkpoint inhibition in metastatic gastric cancer. Annals of Oncology. 2019;**30**:424-430

[24] Zhang B, Wu Q, Li B, et al. M6A regulator-mediated methylation modification patterns and tumor microenvironment infiltration characterization in gastric cancer. Molecular Cancer. 2020;**19**:53

[25] Li B, Jiang Y, Li G, et al. R, natural killer cell and stroma abundance are independently prognostic and predict gastric cancer chemotherapy benefit. JCI Insight. 2020;**5**:e136570

[26] Hsieh H-L, Tsai M-M. Tumor progression-dependent angiogenesis in gastric cancer and its potential application. World Journal of Gastrointestinal Oncology. 2019;**11**:686-704

[27] Sammarco G, Varricchi G, Ferraro V, et al. Mast cells, angiogenesis and lymphangiogenesis in human gastric cancer. International Journal of Molecular Sciences. 2019;**20**:2106

[28] Feng Y, Dai Y, Gong Z, et al. Association between angiogenesis and cytotoxic signatures in the tumor microenvironment of gastric cancer. Oncotargets and Therapy. 2018;**11**:2725-2733

[29] Huinen ZR, Huijbers EJM, van Beijnum JR, et al. Anti-angiogenic agents – Overcoming tumour endothelial cell energy and improving immunotherapy outcomes. Nature Reviews. Clinical Oncology. 2021;**18**:527-540

[30] Turner N, Grose R. Fibroblast growth factor signalling: From development to cancer. Nature Reviews. Cancer. 2010;**10**:116-129

[31] Lieu C, Heymach J, Overman M, et al. Beyond VEGF: Inhibition of the fibroblast growth factor pathway and antiangiogenesis. Clinical Cancer Research. 2011;**17**:6130-6139

[32] Liu D, Ma X, Yang F, et al. Discovery and validation of methylated-differentially expressed genes in Helicobacter pylori-induced gastric cancer. Cancer Gene Therapy. 2020;**27**(6):473-485

[33] Ciciola P, Cascetta P, Bianco C, et al. Combining immune checkpoint inhibitors with anti-angiogenic agents. Journal of Clinical Medicine. 2020;**9**:675

[34] Haghighi SR, Asadi MH, Akrami H. Anti-carcinogenic and anti-angiogenic properties of the extracts of Acorus calamus on gastric cancer cells. Avicenna Journal of Phytomedicine. 2017;**7**:145

[35] Zhang M, Deng W, Cao X, et al. Concurrent apatinib and local radiation therapy for advanced gastric cancer: A

case report and review of the literature. Medicine. 2017;**96**:e6241

[36] Mawalla B, Yuan X, Luo X, et al. Treatment outcome of anti-angiogenesis through VEGF-pathway in the management of gastric cancer: A systematic review of phase II and III clinical trials. BMC Research Notes. 2018;**11**:21

[37] Lei X, Wang F, Ke Y, et al. The role of antiangiogenic agents in the treatment of gastric cancer: A systematic review and meta-analysis. Medicine. 2017;**96**:e6301

[38] Qin S, Li A, Yi M, et al. Recent advances on anti-angiogenesis receptor tyrosine kinase inhibitors in cancer therapy. Journal of Hematology & Oncology. 2019;**12**:1-11

[39] Qu J, Zhang Y, Chen X, et al. Newly developed anti-angiogenic therapy in non-small cell lung cancer. Oncotarget. 2018;**9**:10147-10163

[40] Bai Z-G, Zhang Z-T. A systematic review and meta-analysis on the effect of angiogenesis blockade for the treatment of gastric cancer. Oncotargets and Therapy. 2018;**11**:7077-7087

[41] Dong M, Wang R, Sun P, et al. Clinical significance of hypertension in patients with different types of cancer treated with antiangiogenic drugs. Oncology Letters. 2021;**21**:315

[42] Miller H, Czigany Z, Lurje I, et al. Impact of angiogenesis- and hypoxia-associated polymorphisms on tumor recurrence in patients with hepatocellular carcinoma undergoing surgical resection. Cancers. 2020;**12**:3826

[43] Zhao Y, Tang Y, Qin H, Feng K, Hu C. The efficient circulating immunoscore predicts prognosis of patients with advanced gastrointestinal cancer. World Journal of Surgical Oncology. 2022;**20**(1):233

[44] Yu X, He S, Shen J, et al. Tumor vessel normalization and immunotherapy in gastric cancer. Therapeutic Advances in Medical Oncology. 2022;**14**:17588359221110176

[45] Lv D, Khawar MB, Liang Z, Gao Y, Sun H. Neoantigens and NK cells: "Trick or treat" the cancers? Frontiers in Immunology. 2022;**13**:931862

[46] Dunn GP, Bruce AT, Ikeda H, Old LJ, Schreiber RD. Cancer Immunoediting: From Immunosurveillance to tumor escape. Nature Immunology. 2002;**3**(11):991-998

[47] Ribatti D. The concept of immune surveillance against tumors. First Theories Oncotarget. 2017;**8**(4):7175-7180

[48] Jhunjhunwala S, Hammer C, Delamarre L. Antigen presentation in cancer: Insights into tumour immunogenicity and immune evasion. Nature Reviews. Cancer. 2021;**21**(5):298-312

[49] Balasubramanian A, John T, Asselin-Labat ML. Regulation of the antigen presentation machinery in cancer and its implication for immune surveillance. Biochemical Society Transactions. 2022;**50**(2):825-837

[50] Rosenberg SA. Il-2: The first effective immunotherapy for human cancer. Journal of Immunology. 2014;**192**(12):5451-5458

[51] Riley RS, June CH, Langer R, Mitchell MJ. Delivery Technologies for Cancer Immunotherapy. Nature Reviews. Drug Discovery. 2019;**18**(3):175-196

[52] Galon J, Bruni D. Approaches to treat immune hot, altered and cold Tumours with combination immunotherapies. Nature Reviews. Drug Discovery. 2019;**18**(3):197-218

[53] Long EO, Kim HS, Liu DF, Peterson ME, Rajagopalan S. Controlling natural killer cell responses: Integration of signals for activation and inhibition. Annual Review of Immunology. 2013;**31**:227-258

[54] Tumeh PC, Harview CL, Yearley JH, et al. Pd-1 blockade induces responses by inhibiting adaptive immune resistance. Nature. 2014;**515**(7528):568-571

[55] Wolchok JD, Chiarion-Sileni V, Gonzalez R, Rutkowski P, Grob JJ, Cowey CL, et al. Overall survival with combined Nivolumab and Ipilimumab in advanced melanoma. The New England Journal of Medicine. 2017;**377**(14):1345-1356

[56] Buchbinder EI, Desai A. Ctla-4 and Pd-1 pathways: Similarities, differences, and implications of their inhibition. American Journal of Clinical Oncology. 2016;**39**(1):98-106

[57] Schmidt C. The benefits of immunotherapy combinations. Nature. 2017;**552**(7685):S67-SS9

[58] Schumacher TN, Scheper W, Kvistborg P. Cancer Neoantigens. Annual Review of Immunology. 2019;**37**:173-200

[59] Smith CC, Selitsky SR, Chai S, Armistead PM, Vincent BG, Serody JS. Alternative tumour-specific antigens. Nature Reviews. Cancer. 2019;**19**(8):465-478

[60] Schumacher TN, Schreiber RD. Neoantigens in cancer immunotherapy. Science. 2015;**348**(6230):69-74

[61] Lu YC, Robbins PF. Cancer immunotherapy targeting Neoantigens. Seminars in Immunology. 2016;**28**(1):22-27

[62] Peng M, Mo Y, Wang Y, et al. Neoantigen vaccine: An emerging tumor immunotherapy. Molecular Cancer. 2019;**18**(1):128

[63] Alexandrov LB, Nik-Zainal S, Wedge DC, et al. Signatures of mutational processes in human cancer. Nature. 2013;**500**(7463):415-421

[64] Turajlic S, Litchfield K, Xu H, et al. Insertion-and-deletion-derived tumour-specific Neoantigens and the immunogenic phenotype: A pan-cancer analysis. The Lancet Oncology. 2017;**18**(8):1009-1021

[65] Yang W, Lee KW, Srivastava RM, et al. Immunogenic Neoantigens derived from gene fusions stimulate T cell responses. Nature Medicine. 2019;**25**(5):767-775

[66] Lang F, Schrors B, Lower M, et al. Identification of Neoantigens for individualized therapeutic cancer vaccines. Nature Reviews. Drug Discovery. 2022;**21**(4):261-282

[67] Coulie PG, Lehmann F, Lethe B, et al. A mutated intron sequence codes for an antigenic peptide recognized by Cytolytic T lymphocytes on a human melanoma. Proceedings of the National Academy of Sciences of the USA. 1995;**92**(17):7976-7980

[68] Wolfel T, Hauer M, Schneider J, et al. A P16ink4a-insensitive Cdk4 mutant targeted by Cytolytic T lymphocytes in a human melanoma. Science. 1995;**269**(5228):1281-1284

[69] Cui C, Wang J, Fagerberg E, et al. Neoantigen-driven B cell and Cd4

T follicular helper cell collaboration promotes anti-tumor Cd8 T cell responses. Cell. 2021;**184**(25):6101-18 e13

[70] Brown SD, Warren RL, Gibb EA, et al. Neo-antigens predicted by tumor genome meta-analysis correlate with increased patient survival. Genome Research. 2014;**24**(5):743-750

[71] Balachandran VP, Luksza M, Zhao JN, et al. Identification of unique Neoantigen qualities in Long-term survivors of pancreatic cancer. Nature. 2017;**551**(7681):512-516

[72] Yamamoto TN, Kishton RJ, Restifo NP. Developing Neoantigen-targeted T cell-based treatments for solid tumors. Nature Medicine. 2019;**25**(10):1488-1499

[73] Hu Z, Ott PA, Wu CJ. Towards personalized, tumour-specific, therapeutic vaccines for cancer. Nature Reviews. Immunology. 2018;**18**(3):168-182

[74] Laskowski TJ, Biederstädt A, Rezvani K. Natural killer cells in antitumour adoptive cell immunotherapy. Nature Reviews. Cancer. 2022;**25**:1-19

Section 3

Natural Killer Cells in Miscarriage

Chapter 4

The Role of NK Cells in Recurrent Miscarriage (Abortion)

Vida Homayouni, Fariba Dehghan and Roya Sherkat

Abstract

Recurrent miscarriage is an early pregnancy complication that affects about 1–3% of couples. There are specific characteristics of natural killer (NK) cells associated with miscarriage. In patients with recurrent miscarriage, a lack of inhibition of decidua natural killer cells can be observed, which leads to a more activated state and presentation of NK cell dim that is characterized by higher levels of pro-inflammatory cytokines and cytotoxicity effect. In peripheral blood, a dysfunctional cytokine production by natural killer cells has been also reported, with an increase of interferon-γ levels and a decrease of interleukin-4. Accordingly, there are different population of NK cells such as dim and bright. The lack of balance between these populations can lead to miscarriage. Using flow cytometry, we can detect these populations and propose the treatment too.

Keywords: abortion, NK cell dim, NK cell bright, recurrent miscarriage, KIR

1. Introduction

Recurrent miscarriage (RM) is an early pregnancy failure that affects about 1–3% of couples who wish to have children [1]. This common complex problem of early pregnancy can be caused etiologically by genetic, anatomical, hormonal, and infectious factors or none etiologic. One underlying cause of unexplained recurrent abortions (RA) may be a maternal immunological factor that causes to interfere with the maternofetal tolerance [2, 3]. Natural killer (NK) cells are important immune cells that participate in innate and adaptive immunity and have roles in recurrent abortion. They include the majority of immune cells present in the maternal-fetal interface. Obviously, uterus and fetus represent immunologically privileged sites and usually, maternal immune system does not attack non-self, paternal inherited, or fetal antigens. The challenge was observed between innate and adaptive immune cells that mediate immune protection at the maternal-fetal interface in immune-privileged sites of the pregnant uterus [4]. Normal fetal growth requires an adequate supply of maternal nutrients and oxygen to the placenta, which is achieved by trophoblast invasion and spiral artery remodeling [5]. NK cells secrete some cytokines and chemokines, such as vasoactive growth factor, placenta growth factor, insulin-like growth factor-binding protein 1 (IGFBP-1), and VEGF to promote this happening [5]. NK cell in peripheral blood and uterus of women with RM have different populations and higher percentage compared with healthy individuals. Indeed, the different expressions of receptors modulate the cytolytic or immunoregulatory condition [6].

2. The receptors of NK cells in abortion

Several factors such as NK cell receptors, cytokines, and hormones, for example, progesterone are involved in successful pregnancy [7]. A successful implantation requires an accurate balance between activation and inhibition of NK cells that are mediated by some receptors including inhibitory and activatory roles. Moreover, a number of receptors are identified as diagnostic markers.

NK cells are lymphocytes that are defined as CD3 − CD56+ population. Peripheral NK (pNK) cells are phenotypically and functionally different from uterine NK (uNK) cells and < 10% of pNK cells are similar to uNK cells. Depending on the intensity of the CD56+ neural cell adhesion molecule, they are classically divided into CD56bright (high intensity, composed of cooperative and tolerogenic cells) and CD56dim (low intensity, more cytotoxic against tumors or virus-infected cells) NK cells.

A subset of the CD56dim NK cell expresses a high level of CD16 (FcγRIII) as a receptor involved in antibody-dependent cell cytotoxicity (ADCC). These are defined by its cytotoxicity function. In contrast, CD56bright NK cells are lack of CD16 and characterized by the production of immune-regulatory cytokines. These are highly proliferative activities. Furthermore, 90% of pNK cells are CD56dim and CD16+, whereas 80% of uNK cells are CD56bright and CD16 negative [8]. CD16 is defined as a unique receptor that functions independently without the help of other receptors of NK cells and acts after the adaptive immune response. The different expressions of receptors modulate the cytolytic or immunoregulatory condition [9]. Some researchers showed a higher percentage of the subpopulation CD56bright NK cells in women who had live births compared with women who miscarried [1]. Furthermore, some studies revealed there are new subpopulations of CD56bright that play a central role in trophoblast interaction. Measuring the ability of NK cytotoxicity or detection of activation markers such as CD69 or CD107a can be identified as predictive value in miscarriage.

In addition, NK activity depends on the activating and inhibitory receptors that are retrieved from several germline-encoded, mainly derived from three families: C-type lectin-like receptors, immunoglobulin (Ig)-like transcripts, and killer cell Ig-like receptors (KIRs). KIRs are classified according to their structure and function. Each KIR molecule consists of two or three extracellular Ig domains (2D and 3D molecules). KIRs are a set of variable gene polymorphisms (each individual inherits 4–20 genes from each parent) that code for inhibitory or activating receptors expressed in a variegated manner on subsets of NK cells and some T cells. Inhibitory and some activating KIR bind to HLA class I molecules, while other activating KIR binds to pathogen components within HLA class I molecules.

3. NK cell and trophoblast

Tolerating the allogeneic fetus by the maternal immune system is essential to a successful pregnancy. In the fetal-maternal interface, the maternal uterine tissue is in direct relation with the fetal-derived trophoblast cells and decidual natural killer (dNK) cells or uterine natural killer (uNK) cells mediate primarily the immune tolerance microenvironment. Uterine natural killer (uNK) cells are a category of NK cells that are located in the uterus and comprise the largest leukocyte population in the endometrium throughout early pregnancy [10]. The maternal tissue contacts with trophoblast cells through paternal antigens [11]. Trophoblast invasion and spiral artery remodeling are responsible for delivering maternal nutrients and oxygen to the

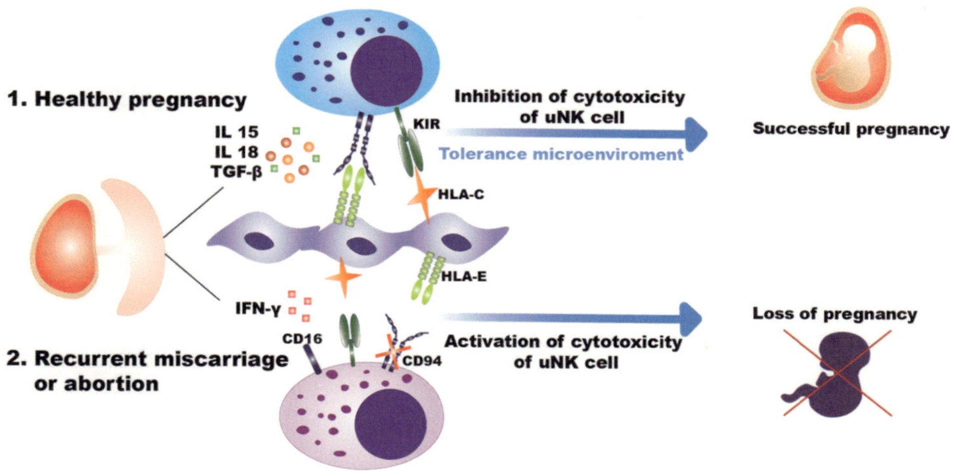

Figure 1.
Difference activation between healthy pregnancy and recurrent miscarriage. The population of NK cells have certain receptors that lead to different function. According to these receptors successful pregnancy or abortion have been happened.

placenta. A major cause of related disorders of pregnancy such as recurrent miscarriage, preeclampsia, and fetal growth restriction is related to diminish trophoblast invasion and vascular reconstruction and it leads to defective placentation [6]. Several studies have revealed that upon interaction with the trophoblast, the activating receptors in dNK cells promote trophoblast invasion and endothelial cell angiogenesis. NK cell secretes cytokines and chemokines such as vasoactive growth factor, placenta growth factor, insulin-like growth factor-binding protein 1 (IGFBP-1), and VEGF. Accordingly, some cytokines such as IL-8, VEGF, SDF-1, and IP-10 and IL-10 promote tolerance microenvironment (**Figure 1**) [7, 12].

4. NK cells are defined as double-edged sword

Peripheral blood NK (pbNK) cells besides playing a substantial role against viral infections and have a tolerogenic role in pregnancy. Unlike most somatic cells that express classical major histocompatibility complex class I (MHC-I) molecules such as HLA-A or HLA-B, trophoblast expresses only some unique HLA class I molecules, including non-classical HLA-E and HLA-G and the only polymorphic class I, for example, HLA-C [13, 14]. Inhibitory dNK cell receptors, such as killer immunoglobulin-like receptors (KIR), interact with specific MHC-I molecules, limiting dNK cell cytotoxicity and helping to maintain the balance of immune tolerance. However, when the intercellular cell-to-cell communication is disrupted at the maternal-fetal interface, insufficient maturation of dNK cells results in decreased immune tolerance and cytotoxic up-regulation (**Figure 2**).

There are numerous mechanisms to influence NK cell immunity by targeting their ligand-receptor, signaling pathways, chemokines, and cytokine secretion in viruses that affect NK cell activation and recruitment. NK cells in turn respond as follows:

1. Recognizing "the missing self" that viruses avoid T-cell responses by downregulating MHC class I.

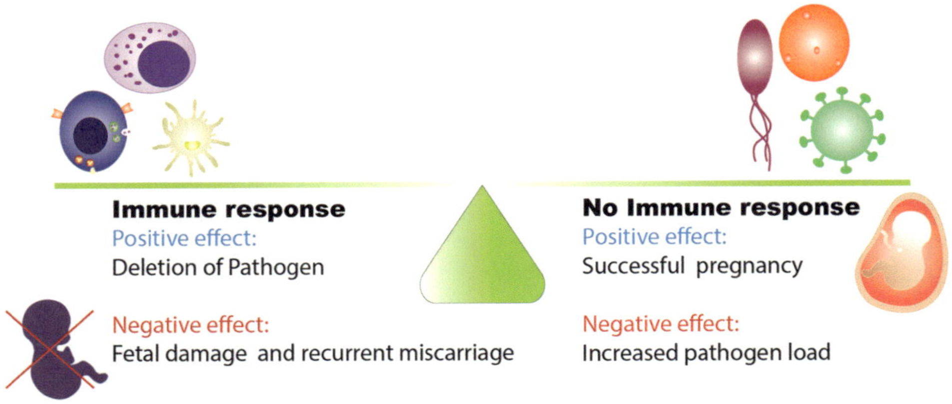

Figure 2.
Immune response behaves as double-edge sword: During pregnancy, the growth of the fetuses and protection from pathogen should be balanced.

2. Recognizing host- and pathogen-derived ligands, by activation of receptors such as NKG2C, NCRs, and NKG2D.

3. Antibody-dependent cytotoxicity by FcγRIII (CD16).

4. Responding to some cytokines such as IL-12, IL-15, and IL-18.

The response to infection in pregnancy was influenced by KIR and HLA variants and depending on these variants dNK cells may eliminate cells infected with pathogens. Some studies revealed that pregnant women with KIR2DS1+ dNK cells activated by ligating with fetal HLA-C2 have a lower chance to exposure pre-eclampsia and increasing the development of placenta. KIR2DL4 is a kind of variant to interact with HLA-G and may have a tolerogenic function. HLA-G can also help infected and cancerous cells escape immune control. Although higher HLA-G levels might modulate the immune response and prevent fetal failure, they can also lead to congenital infections [9].

HLA-E is another molecule that is expressed by trophoblast, maternal leukocytes, and stromal cells, where it interacts with activating CD94/NKG2C and inhibitory CD94/NKG2A, expressed by pbNK and dNK cells. While NKG2C may suppress dNK functions, NKG2A may also promote dNK-cell functions by enhancing NK-cell cytotoxicity [15].

Natural cytotoxicity receptors (NCR) on NK cells include NKp46, NKp30, and NKp44, which regulate host NK cell cytotoxicity and cytokine secretion, as well as pathogen-derived ligands such as hemagglutinin neuraminidases, viral hemagglutinins, and other pathogen components. NKp46, as an NCRs, activates NK cells, while splice variants NKp44 and NKp30 either activate or inhibit. Meanwhile, dNK cells express inhibitory isoforms, and pbNKs express activating isoforms. The switch from activation to inhibition of NKp44 and NKp30 is associated with reduced cytotoxicity and is mediated by exposure of pbNK cells to cytokines present in the decidual environment, such as IL-15, IL-18, and TGF-β. The importance of NKp46 was found in the peripheral blood of women with a history of RM and determined with a decreased percentage of NKp46CD56 bright cells [6].

NKG2D is an activating receptor expressed in the majority of pbNK cells and dNK cells too. It binds ligands induced in stressed cells and therefore alerting immune cells' function. While these ligands are not found on trophoblast, they can be induced on uterine stromal cells and/or produced by trophoblast in soluble forms to interact with both dNK cells and pbNK cells.

T-cell immunoglobulin domain and mucin domain-containing molecule-3 (Tim-3) is a newly defined regulatory factor that can modulate the balance of Th1 cells/Th2 cells and expresses in some dNK cells, and Tim-3+ dNK+ cells displayed decreased cytotoxicity due to producing less perforin [15, 16].

In the non-pregnant endometrium, uterine NK cells (uNK) are largely inactive but have the ability to differentiate and switch to cytotoxic behavior and perform immune defense against intrauterine infection by pathogens [13, 17]. Yan Whua reported the expression of some inhibitory receptors, including KIR2DL4, NKG2A, and KIR2DL1, was significantly lower in women with RM [18, 19]. A high percentage of CD56 + NK cells that expressed KIR specific for HLA-C was observed in healthy women and a decline of this receptor in RM women [14].

5. The cytotoxicity of pNK and uNK cells

The evaluation of uNK cytotoxicity is difficult, rare, and technically challenging. According to a study done by Trundley and Moffett, 2004, we declared that uNK does not possess the same cytotoxic function ability as pNK. In support of this statement, dNK is unable to make activating cytotoxicity signals that trigger perforin release when interacting with classical cancerous target cell lines, such as K562 [20].

The lysis of K562 leukemic cells can be measured after co-incubation with uNK at effector: target (E: T) ratios ranging from 5:1 to 40:1. Percentage of target cell lysis was determined by either a chromium release assay or flow cytometry assay by CFSE method. Indeed, results in uNK cell cytotoxicity case-control studies performed with uNK isolated from first-trimester decidua showed greater target cell lysis in women with RM compared to controls [15]. However, they suggested that there is more pNK in the endometrium of RM patients than in the endometrium of controls. pNK has more ability to kill K562 cancer cells so the accumulation of pNK in the endometrium of RM patients leads to an improvement in the ability of the total number of NK cells to kill K562 cells. In addition, uNK may be more activated in RM patients and thus have increased cytotoxicity function to kill K562 cancer cells, although it cannot result in the same effect also observed in trophoblastic cells.

6. The cytokine expression of pNK and uNK cell

Since uNK derived from women with RM secrete more type 1 cytokine (e.g., IFN-$^{\gamma}$ and TNF-a) compared with type 2 cytokine (e.g., IL-4 and IL-10, TGF-β), the direction of uNK involvement in RM may not be so clear. Moreover, uNK cells are also an important source of angiogenic growth factors, vascular endothelial growth factor (VEGF)-A, VEGF-C, placental growth factor, keratinocyte growth factor, fibroblast growth factor, and platelet-derived growth factor-BB [21].

Although the studies have clinical heterogeneity and differences in the secretory activity of uNK cells, Ledee et al. (2004, 2005, 2008) using a combination of detection assays demonstrated that impairment of vascular remodeling may be caused by either insufficient or excessive NK cell recruitment to the endometrium in addition to dysregulated cytokine signaling. Furthermore, flow cytometry was used as a more objective and robust way which measures the specific antigens CD45 (leucocyte antigen), CD3 (T-cell antigen),

CD56, and CD16 to overcome this source of heterogeneity and perform subgroup analysis. Furthermore, the use of a standardized gating strategy would help to overcome heterogeneity between different studies [22]. Li Zhu et al. have reported a high proportion of circulating activated T lymphocytes, high cytotoxic NK cells, and low population of circulating IL-10 CD56bright NK cells and low IL-4, IL-10, and TGF-β in RM patients [12].

As we mentioned before, some studies revealed there are new subpopulations of CD56bright that play a central role in trophoblast interaction. In humans, dNK1 may engage with trophoblast through KIR. A subset of NKG2C+ dNK1 may provide benefits in secondary pregnancy through immunological development, while dNK2 and dNK3 cells may interact with other cell types in the decidua through the production of other factors such as XCL-1, which can attract both DCs and trophoblast. It is clear that uNK undergoes complex interactions with other cells in the immune milieu of the placental bed along with differentiation to subpopulation. For instance, CD56 + CD94-CD117 + CD127+ type 3 ILC produces IL-22 and IL-8, whereas CD56 + CD94+ ILC-1 may contribute to IFN-$^{\gamma}$ production [23]. This new population of immune cells that are present in the decidua (ILCs) is considered to contribute to producing cytokines pool that interferes in pregnancy. Therefore, more consideration needs to be given to the interaction between uNK and trophoblast cells.

7. Immunotherapy for women with abnormal uNK cell numbers

There are several treatment protocols proposed in literature serving as tools for the management of patients diagnosed with RM that targets the immunological background of these diseases. Proposed treatment options for uNK-related RIF and RM include: Glucocorticoids, Intralipid therapy, Immunoglobulin therapy [15].

7.1 Glucocorticoids

Glucocorticoids could act as anti-inflammatory and immunosuppressant actions. Glucocorticoids have been used to treat women with reproductive failure and high numbers of uNK cells that express the glucocorticoid receptor. This treatment can conduct in the reduction of uNK cell numbers and lead to live birth. They can cause hormonal changes in the fetus. uNK cell-mediated cytotoxicity is sensitive to exogenous glucocorticoids.

7.2 Intralipid therapy

Intralipid is a fat emulsion containing soybean oil, glycerin, and egg phospholipids. Intralipid is used for parenteral nutrition in patients who cannot take food by mouth. The ability of intralipid to suppress the activity of NK cells has been shown in various *in vitro* studies. Animal and human studies illustrate that intravenous intralipid can increase the rate of continued pregnancy by improving implantation in patients with high levels of NK cells. Intralipid may be used as a new effective treatment option for women with RSA and high levels of NK cells [24].

7.3 Immunoglobulin therapy

Intravenous immunoglobulin (IVIg) which is human IgG prepared from pooled plasma administered during pregnancy is used for the treatment of RM. Several theories have been proposed for its action, including the dampening of NK cell number and activity and modification of cytokine production. IVIg therapy in RSA women increases the expression of inhibitory receptor CD94 on NK cells and serum cytokine and shifts the immune system toward Th2 [25]. The underlying mechanism might be associated with the neutralization of autoantibodies, inhibition of natural killer cells, attenuation of cytotoxicity, and increase of regulatory T lymphocytes [26].

7.4 Active immunotherapy (AI) with allogeneic paternal lymphocytes

It appears a feasible treatment option for recurrent abortion (RA). Intradermal immunotherapy with 30–100 million lymphocytes in one to two applications has proven to be effective, associated with low risk, and cost-effective for the treatment of RA. Positive HLA antibody test after AI in RA predicts a successful pregnancy with a probability of 89% making this test suitable as a predictive test [3]. However, the overall response has been followed by severe allergic reactions and painful [27].

8. Conclusion

In this chapter, we reviewed the association between NK cell activity and RM in a number of studies. For instance, a large systematic review published in 2011 was conducted to detect the relationship between NK cell activity and RM. This study showed that the prognostic value of the percentage or activity of peripheral NK cells in patients with idiopathic RSA is still uncertain, and larger studies were recommended. However, a meta-analysis published in 2014 outlined the relationship between peripheral NK cells and RSA by pooling the data from four different studies and found a significant difference in the activity of peripheral NK cells between women with RSA and those in the control group.

Future research should endeavor to reveal single-cell RNA sequencing in first-trimester pregnancies to evaluate pathological pregnancies and immunogenetic screening can be introduced in clinical procedures. Also, the other new population of immune cells that are present in the decidua such as ILCs considered to contribute to the presence of cytokines pool that interfere in pregnancy.

Acknowledgements

We are grateful to the Immunodeficiency Diseases Research Center, and all of those with whom we have had the pleasure to work during this project.

Conflict of interest

We have no conflict of interests to disclose.

Appendices and nomenclature

IDRC	Immunodeficiency Disease Research Center
NK	natural killer cell

RM	recurrent miscarriage
KIR	killer immune receptors
RIF	recurrent implantation failure
ART	assisted reproductive technology

Author details

Vida Homayouni*, Fariba Dehghan and Roya Sherkat
Immunodeficiency Diseases Research Center, Isfahan University of Medical Sciences, Isfahan, Iran

*Address all correspondence to: vidahoma2015@gmail.com

References

[1] Von Woon E, Greer O, Shah N, et al. Number and function of uterine natural killer cells in recurrent miscarriage and implantation failure: A systematic review and meta-analysis. Human Reproduction Update. 2022;**28**:548-582

[2] Shmeleva EV, Colucci F. Maternal natural killer cells at the intersection between reproduction and mucosal immunity. Mucosal Immunology. 2021;**14**:991-1005

[3] Wegener S, Schnurstein K, Hansch S, et al. Immunotherapy with paternal lymphocytes for recurrent miscarriages and unsuccessful in vitro fertilization treatment. Transfusion Medicine and Hemotherapy. 2006;**33**:501-507

[4] Colucci F. The immunological code of pregnancy. Science. 2019;**365**:862-863

[5] Hao F, Zhou X, Jin L. Natural killer cells: Functional differences in recurrent spontaneous abortion. Biology of Reproduction. 2020;**102**:524-531

[6] Guerrero B, Hassouneh F, Delgado E, et al. Natural killer cells in recurrent miscarriage: An overview. Journal of Reproductive Immunology. 2020;**142**:103209. DOI: 10.1016/j.jri.2020.103209

[7] Zhang X, Wei H. Role of Decidual natural killer cells in human pregnancy and related pregnancy complications. Frontiers in Immunology. 2021;**12**:728291. DOI: 10.3389/FIMMU.2021.728291/FULL

[8] Tang AW, Alfirevic Z, Quenby S. Natural killer cells and pregnancy outcomes in women with recurrent miscarriage and infertility: A systematic review. Human Reproduction. 2011;**26**:1971-1980

[9] De Sanctis JB, Garmendia JV, Hajdúch M. Overview of memory NK cells in viral infections: Possible role in SARS-CoV-2 infection. Frontiers in Immunology. 2022;**2**:52-67

[10] Kalkunte S, Chichester CO, Gotsch F, et al. Evolution of non-cytotoxic uterine natural killer cells. American Journal of Reproductive Immunology. 2008;**59**:425-432

[11] Xu L, Li Y, Sang Y, et al. Crosstalk between trophoblasts and Decidual immune cells: The cornerstone of maternal-fetal Immunotolerance. Frontiers in Immunology. 2021;**12**:642392. DOI: 10.3389/fimmu.2021.642392

[12] Zhu L, Aly M, Kuon RJ, et al. Patients with idiopathic recurrent miscarriage have abnormally high TGFß+ blood NK, NKT and T cells in the presence of abnormally low TGFß plasma levels. BMC Immunology. 2019;**20**:10. DOI: 10.1186/S12865-019-0290-3

[13] Tower C, Walker JJ, Mulder A, et al. Maternal activating KIRs protect against human reproductive failure mediated by fetal HLA-C2. The Journal of Clinical Investigation. 2010;**121**:455-455

[14] Faridi RM, Agrawal S. Killer immunoglobulin-like receptors (KIRs) and HLA-C allorecognition patterns implicative of dominant activation of natural killer cells contribute to recurrent miscarriages. Human Reproduction. 2011;**26**:491-497

[15] Sfakianoudis K, Rapani A, Grigoriadis S, et al. The role of uterine

natural killer cells on recurrent miscarriage and recurrent implantation failure: From pathophysiology to treatment. Biomedicine. 2021;**9**:1425. DOI: 10.3390/biomedicines9101425

[16] Kim J, Phan MTT, Kweon SH, et al. A flow cytometry-based whole blood natural killer cell cytotoxicity assay using overnight cytokine activation. Frontiers in Immunology. 2020;**11**:1851. DOI: 10.3389/FIMMU.2020.01851/FULL

[17] Chazara O, Moffett A. Association of maternal KIR and fetal HLA-C genes with the risk of preeclampsia in the Chinese Han population. Placenta. 2015;**36**:967

[18] Hua YW, Lin A, Guo CB, et al. Possible roles of KIR2DL4 expression on uNK cells in human pregnancy. American Journal of Reproductive Immunology. 2007;**57**:233-242

[19] Guo W, Fang L, Li B, et al. Decreased human leukocyte antigen-G expression by miR-133a contributes to impairment of proinvasion and proangiogenesis functions of decidual NK cells. Frontiers in Immunology. 2017;**8**:741. DOI: 10.3389/FIMMU.2017.00741/FULL

[20] Manaster I, Mizrahi S, et al. Endometrial NK cells are special immature cells that await pregnancy. American Association for Immnology. 2008;**181**:1869-1876. DOI: 10.4049/jimmunol.181.3.1869

[21] Liu J, Dong P, Jia N, et al. The expression of intracellular cytokines of decidual natural killer cells in unexplained recurrent pregnancy loss. Journal of Maternal-Fetal and Neonatal Medicine. 2022;**35**:3209-3215

[22] Huhn O, Ivarsson MA, Gardner L, et al. Distinctive phenotypes and functions of innate lymphoid cells in human decidua during early pregnancy. Nature Communications. 2020;**11**:14123. DOI: 10.1038/s41467-019-14123-z

[23] Toth B, Vomstein K, Togawa R, et al. The impact of previous live births on peripheral and uterine natural killer cells in patients with recurrent miscarriage. Reproductive Biology and Endocrinology. 2019;**17**:72. DOI: 10.1186/S12958-019-0514-7

[24] Dakhly DMR, Bayoumi YA, Sharkawy M, et al. Intralipid supplementation in women with recurrent spontaneous abortion and elevated levels of natural killer cells. International Journal of Gynecology & Obstetrics. 2016;**135**:324-327

[25] Yamada H, Takeda M, Maezawa Y, et al. A high dose intravenous immunoglobulin therapy for women with four or more recurrent spontaneous abortions. ISRN Obstetrics and Gynecology. 2012;**2012**:87-90

[26] Wang S-W, Zhong S-Y, Lou L-J, et al. The effect of intravenous immunoglobulin passive immunotherapy on unexplained recurrent spontaneous abortion: A meta-analysis. Reproductive Biomedicine Online. 2016;**33**:720-736. DOI: 10.1016/j.rbmo.2016.08.025

[27] Stricker RB, Steinleitner A, Winger EE. Intravenous immunoglobulin (IVIG) therapy for immunologic abortion. Clinical and Applied Immunology Reviews. 2002;**2**:187-199

Section 4

Natural Killer Cells and Ionizing Radiation

Chapter 5

Immunomodulation of NK Cells under Ionizing Radiation

Chang-Sheng Shao, Xin Yu, Leisheng Zhang, Ya-Hui Wu and Qing Huang

Abstract

Natural killer (NK) cells are the effector lymphocytes of the innate immune system and control many types of tumors and microbial infections. Ionizing radiation (IR) has a pronounced effect on NK cells. However, the role of NK cells in radiotherapy remains elusive. In this chapter, we summarized the direct and indirect effects of ionizing radiation on NK cells. Low doses of ionizing radiation can enhance the toxic effects of NK cells. In contrast, high doses of ionizing radiation will lead to functional impairment of NK cells. In addition, under ionizing radiation, NK cells are also modulated by other immune cells. Overall, combining NK cell therapy and radiation therapy can improve the efficacy of oncology treatment.

Keywords: natural killer cells, ionizing radiation, radiotherapy, immunotherapy, immunomodulation

1. Introduction

Living on Earth, human beings have always been exposed to natural radiation effects from the universe and the subsurface, which naturally trigger radiobiological phenomena. Since the publication of the first research paper on radiation by the German experimental physicist Roentgen in 1895, research on the processes and biological effects of ionizing radiation has attracted increasing research attention [1]. Ionizing radiation is often used to treat tumors due to its effect on killing tumor cells and is one of the top three current cancer treatments [2]. Ionizing radiation has direct effects on DNA, subcellular organelles, and protein macromolecules in cells, and also has indirect effects on cells by oxidative stress, such as re-damaging DNA by free radicals and damage to the electron respiratory chain [3]. In recent decades, there has been a growing awareness of the interactions between ionizing radiation and the immune system. For a long time, high doses of ionizing radiation were considered to be a net immunosuppression, mainly due to the sensitivity of the lymphatic system to radiation. However, in recent years, studies have increasingly shown that irradiation of local tumors can modulate the immunogenicity of tumor cells and the anti-tumor immune response at the topical and systemic levels of the tumor microenvironment, and in particular, low-dose ionizing radiation can stimulate the cytotoxicity of T and NK cells [4]. Natural killer (NK) cells, which are innate lymphocytes, are important effectors of tumor immune surveillance and play an important role in regulating adaptive immune responses [5]. Ionizing radiation has a significant effect on altering NK cell biology. In addition, we briefly described the importance of ionizing radiation research and summarized its direct and indirect effects on NK cells and the advantages of radiotherapy in combination with immunotherapy.

2. Definition and classification of ionizing radiation

Since Roentgen won the first Nobel Prize in Physics in 1901 for the discovery of X-rays, there has been an exponential increase in the understanding and study of radiation [6, 7]. The discovery of radiation has even driven progress in physics and other scientific fields since the twentieth century. It has had a huge impact on the advancement of science and technology and has become a model research tool and instrument. Radiation is defined in physics as the emission or propagation of energy in the form of particles or waves through space or a medium [8]. Radiation is essentially energy and takes different forms.

Electromagnetic radiation has wave-particle duality, and its nature is an electromagnetic wave. Maxwell used a system of equations to derive electromagnetic waves and predicted that light is an electromagnetic wave [9]. Electromagnetic radiation is distinguished according to frequency or wavelength [10]. All electromagnetic radiation has the same speed, and if the wavelength is shorter and the frequency is higher, the energy is greater, and the energy possessed to pass through the matter is greater. Among them, gamma rays are more energetic than X-rays, which are composed of photons outside the nucleus, while X-rays are composed of photons inside the nucleus.

Particle radiation, also known as particle beams, is the process by which particles that make up matter and move at high speeds, or nucleus made up of elementary particles, transfer energy to other matter by losing their own kinetic energy. Common

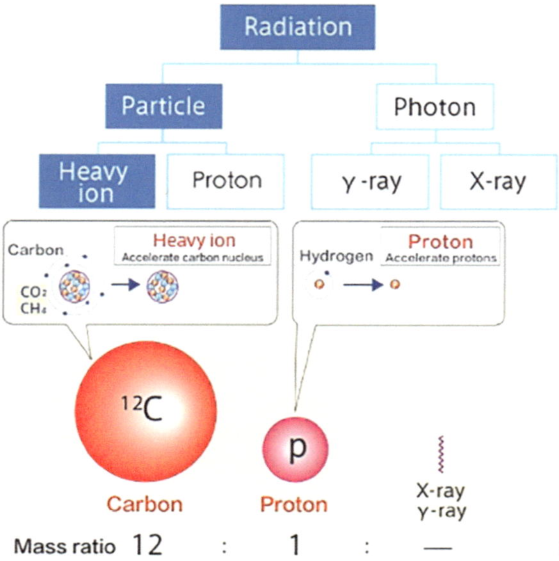

Figure 1.
Commonly used ionizing radiation modalities in clinical practice.

particles are helium nucleus (alpha particles), beta particles, neutrons, protons, heavy ions, etc.

But whether it is particles (α, β, neutrons, protons, charged heavy ions, etc.) or electromagnetic waves (γ-rays, X-rays, etc.), they are ionizing radiation if their energy is sufficient for ionization to occur [11]. As shown in **Figure 1**, the main means of ionizing radiation currently used in clinical practice to treat tumors include photon rays (X-rays, γ-rays) and particle radiation (protons, carbon 12 heavy ions, etc.).

3. Biological effects induced by ionizing radiation

Ionizing radiation can cause direct DNA damage to cells and subcellular organelles (mitochondria, etc.), commonly referred to as target effects.

The direct effects of ionizing radiation on DNA include (1) altering the chemical nature of nucleotides, (2) disrupting the sugar-phosphate backbone, and (3) breaking the hydrogen bonds between bases. Among them, altering the chemical nature of nucleotides is the factor that leads to their mutation [12]. In comparison disruption of the DNA backbone and disruption of hydrogen bonds between bases are physical damages that alter the chemical structure of the DNA molecule [13].

The ionizing radiation-induced DNA damage response is a continuous multilevel response network. The DNA damage signaling process under ionizing radiation is complex. Likewise, it is regulated by a combination of DNA damage signal sensor, apical kinase, damage signal mediator, and downstream kinase [14]. The radiation effects of these early processes further produce beneficial biological effects such as inhibition of cell cycle progression, activation of DNA repair, and maintenance of genomic stability to rescue cells. In contrast, in some cell types or when damage is beyond repair, the reverse effect is initiated, which not only initiates permanent cell cycle arrest (cellular senescence) but also eliminates unrepairable cells by way of programmed cell death [15].

Ionizing radiation also affects DNA indirectly, as mentioned before, ionizing radiation acting on water molecules produces hydrogen (H+) and hydroxyl (OH-) ions. These are called free radicals, as shown in **Figure 2**. Since free radicals are highly reactive, they can easily bind to other ions within the cell. For example, hydroxyl ions (OH-) can react with hydrogen atoms within DNA molecules to form hydrogen peroxide (H_2O_2), which can continue to cause DNA damage, and free radicals can accumulate to cause ongoing damage [16]. Free radical damage is associated with diseases such as aging, cancer, and Alzheimer's disease. Studies have shown that about 65% of cell death caused by ionizing radiation is generated by DNA breakage damage caused by hydroxyl radicals (-OH) [17, 18].

In addition, ionizing radiation can produce bystander effects on cells. As early as 1954, a study reported that plasma from patients treated with local radiation-induced chromosomal aberrations in lymphocytes from patients not treated with radiation, which is one of the most classic cases of bystander effects [19]. In general, paracrine effects are those in which irradiated cells (by alpha particles, X-rays or gamma rays, heavy ions, etc.) can release a certain number of signaling molecules. These signaling molecules are transferred through media or gap junctions, consequently, cytotoxicity or genotoxicity can be observed in non-irradiated cells [20–22].

The mechanism of the paracrine effect may be a signaling pathway, such as the irradiated cell releasing an "attack" signal that is transmitted to distant cells and attacks neighboring cells or diffusion through cellular gap-junction intercellular

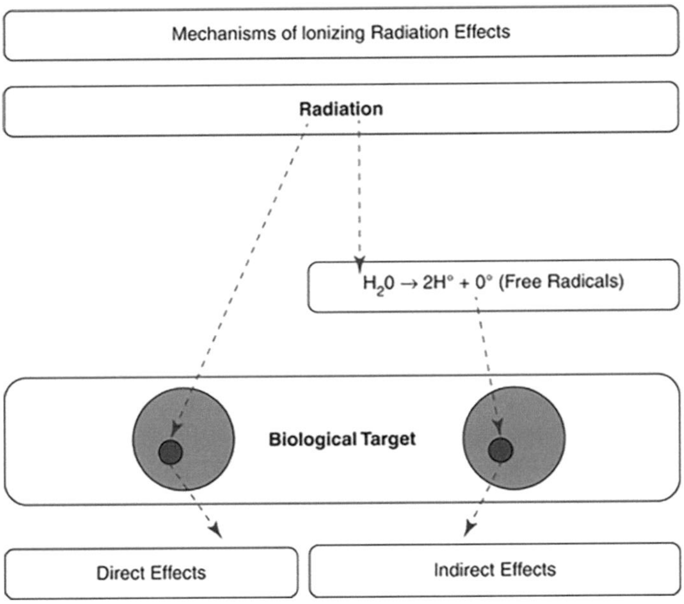

Figure 2.
Direct and indirect effects of ionizing radiation on the cells [13].

communication (Gap-junction) or through certain media. The generation release, and propagation of these signals, such as free radicals and reactive oxygen species generated by ionizing radiation, play a vital role in bystander effects [23, 24]. In addition, some signal transduction pathways may be associated with side effects caused by ionizing radiation, such as MAPK pathway, NO signaling pathway, interleukins (IL-1, IL-8), etc. [25].

Ionizing radiation leads to many forms of cellular processes and effects. These include but are not limited to apoptosis, necrosis, necroptosis, autophagy, and autophagic death. In addition, ionizing radiation can likewise have biological effects on immune cells.

4. The effects of ionizing radiation on NK cells

Ionizing radiation induces immune death of tumor cells, leading to the release of tumor antigens and damage-associated molecular patterns (DAMPs), which in turn stimulate and activate antigen-presenting cells (e.g., dendritic cells and T cells). The above processes can lead to the proliferation of cytotoxic T cells (CTLs), which then migrate into the tumor and initiate an anti-tumor immune response. In addition, ionizing radiation also affects tumor-associated macrophages (TAMs). Ionizing radiation induces macrophage infiltration and differentiation in tumors. Moreover, ionizing radiation promotes the activation of pro-inflammatory macrophages (M2) and enhances their immunostimulatory and tumoricidal activities (**Figure 3**). A growing number of studies now show that ionizing radiation may modulate the function of other innate immune cells, such as myeloid-derived suppressor cells, NK cells, tumor-associated neutrophils, and other cell types [26].

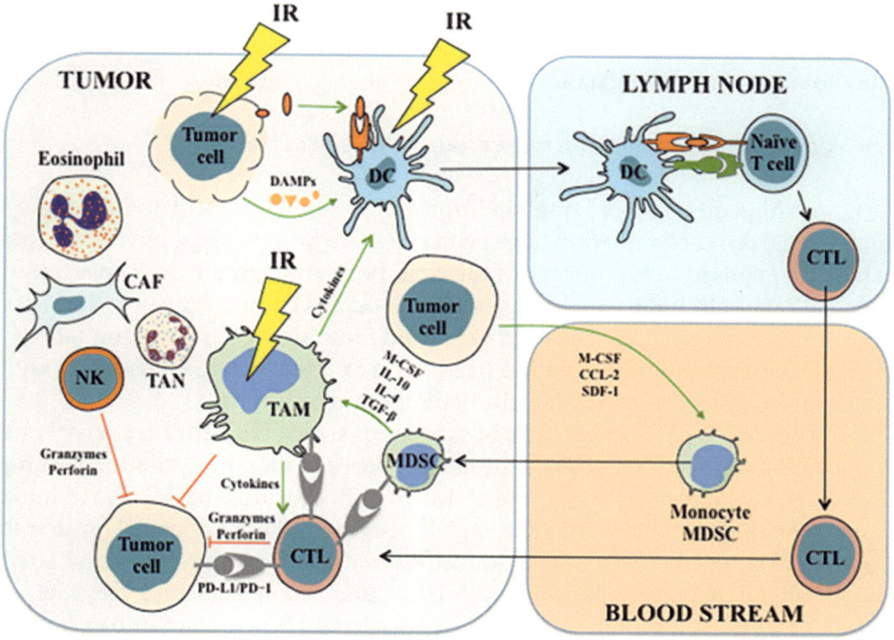

Figure 3.
Schematic diagram of the pathway of the effect of ionizing radiation on immune cells [26].

NK cells play a key role in anti-tumor immunity [27, 28]. NK cells are phenotypically determined by the expression of CD56 and the absence of CD3 and can be classically divided into two populations: CD56bright CD16dim population and CD56dim CD16bright population. Irradiation can directly affect the function of NK cells.

The effect of ionizing irradiation on the function of NK cells was significant. In vitro studies have shown that X-ray irradiation from 5 to 15 Gy doses can temporarily increase the activity of NK cells [29, 30]. The cytotoxic activity of human peripheral blood NK cells was reported to be enhanced at an irradiation dose of 1 Gy, reaching a maximum at 6 Gy. In addition, low-dose gamma irradiation at less than 0.2 Gy induced NK cell expansion and enhanced NK cell cytotoxicity [31]. Low-dose ionizing radiation significantly increased the expression of IFN-γ and TNF-α in NK cells in a p38MAPK-dependent manner [32]. Ionizing irradiation can also affect NK cell function by modulating the interaction between tumor cells and NK cells. For example, ionizing irradiation can upregulate the expression of natural-killer group 2, member D (NKG2D) ligand, and HSP70 in tumor cells, which may increase the sensitivity of tumor cells to NK cell-mediated cytolytic attack [33, 34].

It is still controversial that high and low doses of ionizing radiation have different effects on NK cell function. Rana et al. found that exposure of peripheral blood mononuclear cells to different doses of gamma radiation increased the sensitivity of human NK cell activity (binding and killing). Peripheral blood mononuclear cells were irradiated with low (2–6 Gy) and high (10–30 Gy) doses, and NK cell binding and cytotoxic activity against K562 target cells were studied after 3 and 48 hours of incubation. An overall decrease in cytotoxic activity was observed, but ionizing radiation produced a selected subpopulation of more cytotoxic NK cells and thus may be considered more resistant to radiation damage than the less cytotoxic NK cells [35]. Vokurková et al. identified the secondary CD8+ subpopulation of NK cells as a radiosensitive lymphocyte population whose disappearance was directly correlated with the dose received. Thus, CD3−/CD8+ NK cell subpopulations can be used as low-dose bioassay markers [36, 37].

4.1 Low-dose ionizing radiation can enhance NK cell activity

Although high doses of ionizing radiation are generally harmful and damaging to organisms, low doses of radiation have been shown to be beneficial in various animal models. Mice exposed to low doses of radiation, both very low and low doses, exhibited normal ranges of body weight and whole blood cell counts. However, increased levels of cytokine release in serum and exhibited inhibition of pro-inflammatory responses [38]. Shin et al. showed that irradiation of mice with low doses (0.1 Gy) of X-rays significantly stimulated NK cell-mediated tumor cell lysis [39].

Since NK cells are early responders to exogenous stress, NK cells may reveal rapid subtle changes in function after exposure to low doses of ionizing radiation. Sonn et al. demonstrated that low doses (dose rate of 4.2 mGy/h, total dose of 0.2 Gy) of ionizing radiation promoted anti-tumor toxicity in NK cells but did not affect cell proliferation or apoptosis [31]. Then what would be the effect on NK cells if they were irradiated at a much lower dose? Lacoste et al. further irradiated 560 mice using a very low dose (10 cGy/year) and found that ultra-low dose irradiation did not impair immune system damage by examining mouse lifespan and immune response effects [40].

However, because the mechanism by which low-dose ionizing radiation enhances NK killing is unclear, a great deal of exploration and research has been conducted. Yoon et al. found that low-dose ionizing radiation not only increased the expression of chemokines in tumor cells, but more importantly, increased the expression of CXCL16 (ligand of CXCR6) in NK cells. The above findings suggest that low-dose ionizing radiation enhances the migration of NK cells to tumor sites and achieves effective tumor treatment [41]. In addition, low-dose irradiation has been reported to increase NKG2D ligand expression and enhance NK toxicity [42]. Several studies have claimed that low-dose ionizing radiation may induce direct expansion and activation of NK cells via the P38-MAPK pathway, providing a potential mechanism for low-dose radiation stimulation of NK cells and a novel but simplified stimulation method for NK cell pericyte therapy [32]. Ionizing radiation also triggers the release of a second mitochondria-derived caspase activator (Smac) that competes with X-linked inhibitory apoptosis proteins to enhance NK cell-mediated apoptosis of tumor cells [43]. Currently, in response to heat shock proteins that increase apoptotic resistance of tumor cells, some studies have found that the combination of quercetin and low-dose irradiation can be used to decrease the expression of heat shock protein HSP70, increase the expression of NKG2D, and improve the killing ability of NK cells [44].

4.2 High-dose radiation impairs NK cell immunity

Many treatments directly and adversely affect NK cell function, but observations obtained through in vitro systems may differ from those obtained using clinical samples. Radiotherapy affects NK cell antitumor immunity from multiple perspectives, and the interactions are complex [45]. Radiotherapy produces non-targeted effects on normal tissues such as bone marrow. Thus, alteration of the microenvironment by ionizing radiation is thought to affect the dynamic host-cancer ecosystem, thus influencing cancer behavior including metastasis. Shin et al. demonstrated that high doses of irradiation in mice result in progressive depletion of total leukocytes and platelets at a later stage, with the highest number of NK cells in lung tissue. Thus high doses of radiation can cause hematotoxicity and lung metastasis [46]. p53 tumor suppressor gene has been shown to be associated with programmed cell death, apoptosis in immature thymocytes of mice after ionizing radiation treatment, as reported by Seki et al. High-dose ionizing radiation also induces apoptotic cell death in peripheral mature lymphocytes [47].

In addition, it has also been reported that ionizing radiation may produce adverse reactions and promote tumor metastasis. Heo et al. found that ionizing radiation induces the expression of matrix metalloproteinases (MMPs), which play an important role in the invasion and metastasis of cancer cells. While MMPs have been shown to increase the shedding of NKG2DLs, which may decrease the surface expression of NKG2DLs on cancer cells. Therefore, cancer cells may evade NK-mediated anticancer immunity due to ionizing radiation intervention [48].

5. Combination of ionizing radiation and immunotherapy for anti-tumor

Radioresistance is a major challenge in the treatment of NK/T-cell lymphoma. Wu et al. found that miR-150 was significantly reduced in NK/T-cell lymphoma tissues and cell lines by analyzing a large number of clinical samples. Low miR-150 expression was positively correlated with treatment resistance, and overexpression of miR-150 inhibited the PI3K/AKT/mTOR pathway, thereby significantly enhancing the sensitivity of NK/T-cell lymphoma cells to ionizing radiation therapy [49].

Rational combination therapeutic strategies have been shown to be beneficial in the management of cancer. Regulatory T (T reg) cells are densely distributed in solid tumors, which may promote progression by suppressing anti-tumor immune responses. Bos et al. found that short-term ablation of T reg cells in advanced spontaneous tumors leads to extensive apoptotic tumor cell death. This anti-tumor activity was dependent on IFN-γ and CD4+ T cells, but not on NK or CD8+ T cells. Transient regulatory T cell ablation blocks oncogene-driven breast cancer and provides overall survival by increasing tumor killing in combination with ionizing radiation [50]. Jeong et al. showed that ionizing irradiation enhanced the adhesion between NK cells and target cells by upregulating intercellular adhesion molecule-1 (ICAM-1) on target cells. Ionizing irradiation upregulated ICAM-1 expression on the surface of human cancer cells and enhanced activated NK cell-mediated cytotoxicity. Thus, this also provides a basis for the possibility that ionizing irradiation combined with NK cell therapy may enhance the antitumor effects of NK cells [51].

In addition, ionizing radiation can be combined with mild heat therapy for anti-tumor enhancement of NK cell immune response. Recent studies have shown that the application of local thermotherapy in combination with standard oncologic therapies such as radiotherapy and/or chemotherapy may not only improve local tumor control but also lead to systemic and immune-mediated anti-tumor responses. Werthmöller et al. reported that a local irradiation and heating procedure was established in a mouse model of melanoma and found that tumors treated with ionizing irradiation and heat therapy had significantly delayed tumor growth compared to tumors treated with radiotherapy alone. This combined treatment produced a beneficial tumor microenvironment by enhancing infiltration of CD11c+/MHCII+/CD86+ dendritic cells, CD8+ T cells, and NK cells, and reduced regulatory T cells and myeloid-derived suppressor cells [52]. Thus, ionizing radiation combined with heat therapy has the potential to lead to immunostimulation of anti-tumor immunity.

6. Conclusion

As a complement to antitumor T-cell immunity, NK cells are independent of antigen presentation and can kill tumors directly in a major histocompatibility complex (MHC)-independent manner. A large number of engineered modified NK cell therapies are now proposed, with particular emphasis on anti-tumor immunotherapy. This chapter focuses on the functional changes in NK cells caused by different doses of ionizing radiation are essential. Low doses of ionizing radiation can enhance the toxic effects of NK cells. On the contrary, high doses of ionizing radiation will lead to functional impairment of NK cells. In addition, the combined application of radiotherapy and immunotherapy in clinical treatment is also highly promising.

However, the involved mechanisms are still largely unexplored. With the elucidation of the molecular basis of NK cells activated by proper ionizing radiation, radiation therapy may be better applied with the facilitation of the modulation of the immune system.

Funding

This work was supported by the National Natural Science Foundation of China (Grant No. 11635013, 82260031), the project Youth Fund supported by Shandong Provincial Natural Science Foundation (ZR2020QC097), Science and technology projects of Guizhou Province (QKH-J-ZK[2021]-107), Natural Science Foundation of Jiangxi Province (20224BAB206077, 20212BAB216073), Key Project funded by Department of Science and Technology of Shangrao City (2020AB002, 2022AB003), the Non-profit Central Research Institute Fund of Chinese Academy of Medical Sciences (2019PT320005), and the 2021 Central-Guided Local Science and Technology Development Fund (ZYYDDFFZZZJ-1).

Conflict of interest

The authors declare no conflict of interest.

Author details

Chang-Sheng Shao[1], Xin Yu[2,3], Leisheng Zhang[2,4]*, Ya-Hui Wu[2,3] and Qing Huang[2]*

1 CAS High Magnetic Field Laboratory, Hefei Institutes of Physical Science, Chinese Academy of Sciences, Hefei, China

2 CAS Key Laboratory of High Magnetic Field and Ion Beam Physical Biology, Institute of Intelligent Machines, Hefei Institutes of Physical Science, Chinese Academy of Sciences, Hefei, China

3 Science Island Branch of Graduate School, University of Science and Technology of China, Hefei, China

4 Key Laboratory of Molecular Diagnostics and Precision Medicine for Surgical Oncology in Gansu Province & NHC Key Laboratory of Diagnosis and Therapy of Gastrointestinal Tumor, Gansu Provincial Hospital, China

*Address all correspondence to: leisheng_zhang@163.com and huangq@ipp.ac.cn

References

[1] Behling R. X-ray sources: 125 years of developments of this intriguing technology. Physica Medica. 2020;**79**:162-187

[2] Deng L, Liang H, Fu S, Weichselbaum RR, Fu Y-X. From DNA damage to nucleic acid sensing: A strategy to enhance radiation therapy. Clinical Cancer Research. 2016;**22**(1):20-25

[3] Trachootham D, Alexandre J, Huang P. Targeting cancer cells by ROS-mediated mechanisms: A radical therapeutic approach? Nature Reviews. Drug Discovery. 2009;**8**(7):579-591

[4] Frey B, Rückert M, Deloch L, Rühle PF, Derer A, Fietkau R, et al. Immunomodulation by ionizing radiation—impact for design of radio-immunotherapies and for treatment of inflammatory diseases. Immunological Reviews. 2017;**280**(1):231-248

[5] Artis D, Spits H. The biology of innate lymphoid cells. Nature. 2015;**517**(7534):293-301

[6] Nordlund K, Zinkle SJ, Sand AE, Granberg F, Averback RS, Stoller RE, et al. Primary radiation damage: A review of current understanding and models. Journal of Nuclear Materials. 2018;**512**:450-479

[7] Wessels BW, Buchsbaum DJ. Dosimetry of radiolabeled antibodies. In: Smith AR, editor. Radiation Therapy Physics. Berlin, Heidelberg: Springer Berlin Heidelberg; 1995. pp. 365-384

[8] Jackson SP, Bartek J. The DNA-damage response in human biology and disease. Nature. 2009;**461**(7267):1071-1078

[9] Sengupta DL, Sarkar TK. Maxwell, Hertz, the Maxwellians, and the early history of electromagnetic waves. In: IEEE Antennas and Propagation Magazine. Vol. 45, No. 2; Apr 2003. pp. 13-19. DOI: 10.1109/MAP.2003.1203114

[10] Shao C-S, Zhou X-H, Miao Y-H, Wang P, Zhang Q-Q, Huang Q. In situ observation of mitochondrial biogenesis as the early event of apoptosis. iScience. 2021;**24**(9):103038

[11] Yusof N, Hilmy N. Radiation biology of tissue radiosterilization. 2014:263-287

[12] Lei G, Zhang Y, Koppula P, Liu X, Zhang J, Lin SH, et al. The role of ferroptosis in ionizing radiation-induced cell death and tumor suppression. Cell Research. 2020;**30**(2):146-162

[13] Elgazzar AH, Kazem N. Biological effects of ionizing radiation. 2014:715-726

[14] Vaddavalli PL, Schumacher B. The p53 network: Cellular and systemic DNA damage responses in cancer and aging. Trends in Genetics. 2022;**38**(6):598-612

[15] Khanna KK, Jackson SP. DNA double-strand breaks: Signaling, repair and the cancer connection. Nature Genetics. 2001;**27**(3):247-254

[16] Guleria R. Harmful effects of ionizing radiation. International Journal for Research in Applied Science and Engineering Technology. 2019;**7**(12):887-889

[17] Dizdaroglu M, Jaruga P. Mechanisms of free radical-induced damage to DNA. Free Radical Research. 2012;**46**(4):382-419

[18] Cadet J, Delatour T, Douki T, Gasparutto D, Pouget J-P, Ravanat J-L,

et al. Hydroxyl radicals and DNA base damage. Mutation Research, Fundamental and Molecular Mechanisms of Mutagenesis. 1999;**424**(1-2):9-21

[19] Mothersill C, Seymour C. Radiation-induced bystander effects: Past history and future directions. Radiation Research. 2001;**155**(6):759-767

[20] Heeran AB, Berrigan HP, O'Sullivan J. The radiation-induced bystander effect (RIBE) and its connections with the hallmarks of cancer. Radiation Research. 2019;**192**(6):668-679

[21] Silva PFL, Ogrodnik M, Kucheryavenko O, Glibert J, Miwa S, Cameron K, et al. The bystander effect contributes to the accumulation of senescent cells in vivo. Aging Cell. 2019;**18**(1):e12848

[22] Seymour C, Mothersill C. Cell communication and the "bystander effect". Radiation Research. 1999;**151**(4):505

[23] Morgan WF, Sowa MB. Non-targeted bystander effects induced by ionizing radiation. Mutation Research, Fundamental and Molecular Mechanisms of Mutagenesis. 2007;**616**(1-2):159-164

[24] Prise KM, O'Sullivan JM. Radiation-induced bystander signalling in cancer therapy. Nature Reviews. Cancer. 2009;**9**(5):351-360

[25] Daguenet E, Louati S, Wozny A-S, Vial N, Gras M, Guy J-B, et al. Radiation-induced bystander and abscopal effects: Important lessons from preclinical models. British Journal of Cancer. 2020;**123**(3):339-348

[26] Wu Q, Allouch A, Martins I, Brenner C, Modjtahedi N, Deutsch E, et al. Modulating both tumor cell death and innate immunity is essential for improving radiation therapy effectiveness. Frontiers in Immunology. 2017;**8**:613

[27] Smyth MJ, Cretney E, Kelly JM, Westwood JA, Street SEA, Yagita H, et al. Activation of NK cell cytotoxicity. Molecular Immunology. 2005;**42**(4):501-510

[28] Myers JA, Miller JS. Exploring the NK cell platform for cancer immunotherapy. Nature Reviews. Clinical Oncology. 2021;**18**(2):85-100

[29] Uchida A, Mizutani Y, Nagamuta M, Ikenaga M. Effects of X-ray irradiation on natural killer (NK) cell system. I. Elevation of sensitivity of tumor cells and lytic function of NK cells. Immunopharmacology and Immunotoxicology. 1989;**11**(2-3):507-519

[30] Sakamoto N, Ishikawa T, Kokura S, Okayama T, Oka K, Ideno M, et al. Phase I clinical trial of autologous NK cell therapy using novel expansion method in patients with advanced digestive cancer. Journal of Translational Medicine. 2015;**13**(1):277

[31] Sonn CH, Choi JR, Kim T-J, Yu Y-B, Kim K, Shin SC, et al. Augmentation of natural cytotoxicity by chronic low-dose ionizing radiation in murine natural killer cells primed by IL-2. Journal of Radiation Research. 2012;**53**(6):823-829

[32] Yang G, Kong Q, Wang G, Jin H, Zhou L, Yu D, et al. Low-dose ionizing radiation induces direct activation of natural killer cells and provides a novel approach for adoptive cellular immunotherapy. Cancer Biotherapy & Radiopharmaceuticals. 2014;**29**(10):428-434

[33] Gehrmann M, Marienhagen J, Eichholtz-Wirth H, Fritz E, Ellwart J, Jäättelä M, et al. Dual function of membrane-bound heat shock

protein 70 (Hsp70), Bag-4, and Hsp40: Protection against radiation-induced effects and target structure for natural killer cells. Cell Death and Differentiation. 2005;**12**(1):38-51

[34] Kim J-Y, Son Y-O, Park S-W, Bae J-H, Chung JS, Kim HH, et al. Increase of NKG2D ligands and sensitivity to NK cell-mediated cytotoxicity of tumor cells by heat shock and ionizing radiation. Experimental & Molecular Medicine. 2006;**38**(5):474-484

[35] Rana R, Vitale M, Mazzotti G, Manzoli L, Papa S. Radiosensitivity of human natural killer cells: Binding and cytotoxic activities of natural killer cell subsets. Radiation Research. 1990;**124**(1):96

[36] Vokurková D, Šinkora J, Vávrová J, Řezáčová M, Knížek J, Östereicher J. CD8+ natural killer cells have a potential of a sensitive and reliable biodosimetric marker in vitro. Physiological Research. 2006;**55**(6):689-698

[37] Vokurková D, Vávrová J, Šinkora J, Stoklasová A, Bláha V, Řezáčová M. Radiosensitivity of CD3−CD8+CD56+ NK cells. Radiation Measurements. 2010;**45**(9):1020-1023

[38] Janiak MK, Wargocka JW, Cheda A, Nowosielska EM, Lisiak E, Bilski M. Modulation of anti-tumour functions of NK cells and macrophages after single low-level exposures of mice to X-rays. International Journal of Low Radiation. 2006;**3**(2/3):178

[39] Shin SC, Lee K-M, Kang YM, Kim K, Kim CS, Yang KH, et al. Alteration of cytokine profiles in mice exposed to chronic low-dose ionizing radiation. Biochemical and Biophysical Research Communications. 2010;**397**(4):644-649

[40] Lacoste-Collin L, Jozan S, Cances-Lauwers V, Pipy B, Gasset G, Caratero C, et al. Effect of continuous irradiation with a very low dose of gamma rays on life span and the immune system in SJL mice prone to B-cell lymphoma. Radiation Research. 2007;**168**(6):725-732

[41] Yoon MS, Pham CT, Phan M-TT, Shin D-J, Jang Y-Y, Park M-H, et al. Irradiation of breast cancer cells enhances CXCL16 ligand expression and induces the migration of natural killer cells expressing the CXCR6 receptor. Cytotherapy. 2016;**18**(12):1532-1542

[42] Amin PJ, Shankar BS. Sulforaphane induces ROS mediated induction of NKG2D ligands in human cancer cell lines and enhances susceptibility to NK cell mediated lysis. Life Sciences. 2015;**126**:19-27

[43] Yang K-L, Wang Y-S, Chang C-C, Huang S-C, Huang Y-C, Chi M-S, et al. Reciprocal complementation of the tumoricidal effects of radiation and natural killer cells. PLoS One. 2013;**8**(4):e61797

[44] Bae J-H, Kim J-Y, Kim M-J, Chang S-H, Park Y-S, Son C-H, et al. Quercetin enhances susceptibility to NK cell-mediated lysis of tumor cells through induction of NKG2D ligands and suppression of HSP70. Journal of Immunotherapy. 2010;**33**(4):391-401

[45] Rosental B, Appel MY, Yossef R, Hadad U, Brusilovsky M, Porgador A. The effect of chemotherapy/radiotherapy on cancerous pattern recognition by NK cells. Current Medicinal Chemistry. 2012;**19**(12):1780-1791

[46] Shin JW, Son JY, Raghavendran HRB, Chung WK, Kim HG, Park HJ, et al. High-dose ionizing radiation-induced hematotoxicity and metastasis in mice model. Clinical & Experimental Metastasis. 2011;**28**(8):803-810

[47] Seki H, Kanegane H, Iwai K, Konno A, Ohta K, Yachie A, et al. Ionizing radiation induces apoptotic cell death in human TcR-γ/δ+ T and natural killer cells without detectable p53 protein. European Journal of Immunology. 1994;**24**(11):2914-2917

[48] Heo W, Lee YS, Son CH, Yang K, Park YS, Bae J. Radiation-induced matrix metalloproteinases limit natural killer cell-mediated anticancer immunity in NCI-H23 lung cancer cells. Molecular Medicine Reports. 2015;**11**(3):1800-1806

[49] Wu SJ, Chen J, Wu B, Wang YJ, Guo KY. microRNA-150 enhances radiosensitivity by inhibiting the AKT pathway in NK/T cell lymphoma. Journal of Experimental & Clinical Cancer Research. 2018;**37**(1):18

[50] Bos PD, Plitas G, Rudra D, Lee SY, Rudensky AY. Transient regulatory T cell ablation deters oncogene-driven breast cancer and enhances radiotherapy. The Journal of Experimental Medicine. 2013;**210**(11):2435-2466

[51] Jeong J-U, Uong TNT, Chung W-K, Nam T-K, Ahn S-J, Song J-Y, et al. Effect of irradiation-induced intercellular adhesion molecule-1 expression on natural killer cell-mediated cytotoxicity toward human cancer cells. Cytotherapy. 2018;**20**(5):715-727

[52] Werthmöller N, Frey B, Rückert M, Lotter M, Fietkau R, Gaipl US. Combination of ionising radiation with hyperthermia increases the immunogenic potential of B16-F10 melanoma cells in vitro and in vivo. International Journal of Hyperthermia. 2016;**32**(1):23-30